3D PRINTED SCAFFOLDS AND BONE TISSUE REGENERATION

Ashutosh D. Bagde

CONTENTS

LIST OF FIGURE..XI
LIST OF TABLE...XIII
LIST OF ABBREVIATION....................................XV
CHAPTER 1..1
CHAPTER 2..9
CHAPTER 3..33
CHAPTER 4..51
CHAPTER 5..71
CHAPTER 6..87

List of Figure

Chapter 1
Figure 1.1: Types of bone grafting 2
Figure 1.2 Application of Tissue Engineering and Regenerative Medicine (TERM) 4

Chapter 2
Figure 2.1 Components of tissue engineering 10
Figure 2.2 Mechanical properties of biomaterials along with bulk materials for a medical purpose [55] 12
Figure 2.3 Various scaffold fabrication techniques 16
Figure 2.4 Flowchart presenting typical SFF technology 20
Figure 2.5 Stereolithography [99] 21
Figure 2.6 Selective Laser Sintering [99] 22
Figure 2.7 3D Printing [99] 23
Figure 2.8 Fused Deposition Modeling [99] 24

Chapter 3
Figure 3.1 The nomenclature used for scaffold architecture design 37
Figure 3.2 Architecture design parameters for scaffold 38
Figure 3.3 Schematic of steps of finite element analysis 41
Figure 3. 4 Porosity of concerning architecture design of scaffold 42
Figure 3.5 Von Mises stress for different composition: S_1, S_2, S_3, and S_4 for β-TCP: ZrO_2, β-TCP: MgO, β-TCP: Al_2O_3 and β-TCP: HA, respectively. 45
Figure 3.6 Effective Young's modulus Vs. Porosity graph for different composition: S_1, S_2, S_3 and S_4 for β-TCP: ZrO_2, β-TCP: MgO, β-TCP: Al_2O_3 and β-TCP: HA respectively. 48

Chapter 4
Figure 4.1 3D- Bioplotter system 53
Figure 4.2 3D printed TCP: HA scaffold 54
Figure 4. 3 Pore size alteration for desired porosity. 56
Figure 4.4 Compression testing setup 57
Figure 4. 5 Porosity and strength of 3D printed scaffold 62
Figure 4.6 SEM showing the morphology of pore and strand 63

Figure 4.7 XRD profile of raw powder and sample sintered at 1200 ^{0}C in microwave sintering. 64
Figure 4.8 FTIR Spectra for raw powder and sintered powder at 1200 ^{0}C. 64
Figure 4.9 24 and 48-hour cytotoxicity analysis of composite material..........66
Figure 4.10 Degradation contour for biomaterials used in the study 68
Figure 4.11 Drug release profile for all cases...................68

Chapter 5

Figure 5.1 PVA binder solution (1 to 7 Wt % concentration from left to right) 73
Figure 5.2 Convectional heating furnace setup 74
Figure 5.3 Microwave furnace setup 75
Figure 5.4 Compression test setup...................77
Figure 5.5 Applied pressure and binder concentration variation relationship..................78
Figure 5.6 Good pellet condition at particular PVA wt. % in binder 78
Figure 5.7 Mechanical properties representation for convectional sintered material. A) Change in porosity with binder ratio. B) change in the strength of pellet concerning binder formulation and temperature of sintering. C) the best binder formulation observed in all sintering cycles, i.e., 1000, 1100, 1200 0C..................81
Figure 5. 8 Strength and porosity change graph for microwave sintering........81
Figure 5.9 Worth factor projection 82
Figure 5.10 XRD plot for β-TCP + 20% HA 83
Figure 5.11 FTIR spectra for materials...................83
Figure 5.12 (A)24 and (B)48-hour cytotoxicity analysis of composite material sintered at different temperature and process...................86

List of Table

Chapter 1

Table1.1: Pros and cons according to the type of graft [5] 3

Chapter 2

Table 2.1 Features to be considered in scaffold biomaterial 13

Table 2.2 Scaffold design parameters for bone tissue engineering given by Thavornyutikarn et al. [50] 15

Table 2.3 Summary of conventional scaffold fabrication technique 17

Table 2.4 Summary of various drug-carrying material..27

Chapter 3

Table 3.1 Biomaterials and their properties..35

Table 3.2 Young's modulus and Poisson's ratio of matrix (β-TCP) material with other particle reinforced; where Ec & μC are Young's modulus and Poisson's ratio of composite 36

Table 3.3 Orientation angle representation...38

Table 3.4 An example of architecture design 38

Chapter 4

Table 4.1 Printing parameter for biomaterial..54

Table 4.2 Porosity calculation of green scaffold 56

Table 4.3 Parameters studied on the 3D printed sintered scaffold. 61

Chapter 5

Table 5.1 Microwave sintering heating rate and effect on strength.................................79

List of Abbreviation

µSLA	: micro-stereolithographic
3DP	: 3-Dimensional printing
AI	: artificial intelligence
Al_2O_3	: Alumina
AM	: additive manufacturing
ATCC	: American Type Culture Collection
BCC	: Body-Centered Cubic
BMP	: Bone Morphogenic Proteins
BTE	: bone tissue engineering
CAD	: computer-aided design
CAM	: computer-aided manufacturing
CPC	: calcium phosphate cement
CS	: Convectional sintering
DCP	: dicalcium phosphate
DCPD	: dicalcium phosphate dehydrates
DLP	: digital light processing
EGF	: epithelial growth factor
ESB	: European Society for Biomaterials
etc	: Et cetera
FDM	: Fused-Deposition-Modeling
FEA	: finite element analysis
FGF	: fibroblast growth factor
FTIR	: Fourier transform infrared spectroscopy
GA	: Gibson Ashby
GAGs	: glycosaminoglycans
HA	: Hydroxyapatite
HIP	: hot isostatic pressing
HP	: hot pressing
LDM	: Low-temperature deposition manufacturing

MBG	:	mesoporous bioactive glass
MCPM	:	monocalcium phosphate monohydrate
MgO	:	Magnesia
MHDS	:	Multi-head deposition system
MIC	:	minimum inhibitory concentration
MTT	:	[3-(4,5-dimethyl-2-thiazolyl)-2,5-diphenyl- 2H tetrazolium bromide]
MWS	:	microwave sintering
NCCS	:	National Center for Cell Sciences
PAM	:	pressure-assisted microsyringe
PED	:	precision extruding deposition
PGA	:	polyglycolic acid
PLA	:	polylactic acid
PLGA	:	poly-dl-lactic-co- glycolic acid
PLLA	:	Poly-l-lactic acid
PMMA	:	poly (methyl methacrylate)
PPF	:	poly (propylene fumarate)
PVA	:	Polyvinyl alcohol
RBCC	:	Reinforced body-centered Cubic
RGR	:	relative growth rate
RP	:	rapid prototyping
SC	:	Simple Cubic
SEM	:	Scanning Electron Microscopy
SFF	:	solid freeform
SLA	:	Stereolithography
SPS	:	sparks plasma sintering
SSLS	:	surface selective laser sintering
TB	:	tuberculosis
TCP	:	Tricalcium phosphate
TERM	:	Tissue Engineering and Regenerative Medicine
TIPS	:	Thermal-induced phase separation
TPP	:	two-photon polymerization
T_R	:	room temperature
T_s	:	sintering temperature

TSS	: two-stage sintering two-stage sintering
VEGF	: vascular endothelial growth factor
XRD	: X-ray diffractometry
ZrO_2	: Zirconium

CHAPTER 1: INTRODUCTION

1.1 Preamble:

Bone provides the structural integrity to our body besides the other imperative functions, such as protecting vital organs, providing an environment for bone marrow, creating blood cells, and acting as a storage area for minerals, particularly calcium. The repair of skeletal disorders is one of the most challenging goals for surgery and related science and a vital need for our society. Degenerative bone disease is caused by trauma or other bone-related disorders like osteoporosis, osteomyelitis, bone tuberculosis, etc., increasing fracture risk and bone deformation [1]. The repair of bone fractures due to these skeletal disorders generally treated with reconstructing bone using temporary and permanent implants such as screws and plates. The materials and the mechanical properties of these implants are critical aspects. Most implants consist of metallic materials resulting in biocompatibility issues like allergies and biomechanical discontinuities like modulus mismatch, resulting in "stress-shielding." Therefore, in recent years a trend from reconstruction using an implant to regeneration can be observed [2].

Regeneration aims at supporting the self-healing capacities of our bodies. However, the body's self-healing capacities are limited. Mechanical stabilization of the fracture site is one of the requirements for healing. The defect in the order of 2.5 cm or higher seems to have a poor natural regeneration history and usually demarcated as a critical size defect, even if mechanically stabilized, resulting in a non-union [3]. These defects need to be filled with either natural or synthesis grafting medium to enable regeneration [2]. The natural grafting medium includes treatment with autograft (transplant within the same body), Isograft (transplant between identical individuals, e.g., Monozygotic twins), Allograft (transplant within the same species), and Xenograft (transplant between different species) [4]. The implanted bone graft of the desired shape has been occupied from the other source and natural bone composition. Another grafting where the synthetic material is engineered for the tissue of interest is denoted as Alloplast. The kind of grafting has been shown in Figure 1.1. Autograft is considered a gold standard procedure; however, the limited graft availability is a primary concern.

In contrast, immune rejection and disease transfer are prime apprehensions during Allograft and Xenograft. The chances of monozygotic twins' availability in each case are rare and hence mostly not considered grafting medium. The detailed pros and cons of each grafting technique have been reviewed by Lee et al. [5] and discussed in Table 1.1

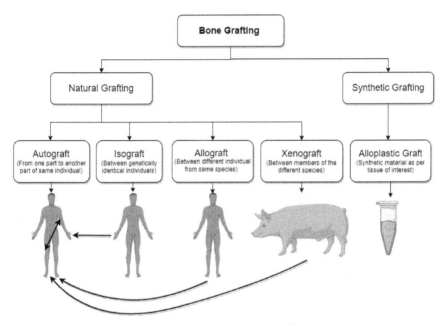

Figure 1.1: Types of bone grafting

The disadvantages of natural grafting give a synthetic grafting medium widespread and broadly covered into Tissue Engineering and Regenerative Medicine (TERM). Tissue engineering is a multidisciplinary field based on elementary principles from biological, chemical, material science, and engineering to repair living tissues using cells, growth factors, mechanical stimuli, and biomaterials. It is inspired by the self-regeneration capability of an organ or tissue. The term tissue engineering was first coined at National Science Foundation Workshop in 1988 to mean 'the application of principles and methods of engineering and life sciences toward the fundamental understanding of structure-function relationships in normal and pathological mammalian tissues and the development of biological substitutes to restore, maintain or improve tissue function [6]. However, the field of tissue engineering may be relatively new; replacing tissue with another goes as far back as the 6th century, as mentioned in *Sushruta Samhita* Fundamental book of Ayurveda describing medicine and surgery). Gasparo Tagliacozzi (1546-99), Professor of Surgery and Anatomy at the University of Bologna in the 16th century, described a nose replacement that he had constructed from a forearm flap in his work 'De Custorum Chirurigia per Insitionem' (The Surgery of Defects by Implantation) was published in 1597 [6]. Langer and Vacanti give the precise definition of tissue engineering in 1993 as "a multidisciplinary scientific branch that combines cell biology, materials science and engineering, and regenerative medicine" [4][7].

Table1.1: Pros and cons according to the type of graft [5]

Type of Graft	Pros	Cons
Autograft	✓ Osteogenesis ✓ Osteoinductive ✓ Osteoconductive ✓ Lack of immunity ✓ No disease transmission ✓ Cost-effective	• Donor site morbidity • Pain • Limited donor site: a limited amount
Allograft	✓ No morbidity of donor site ✓ Unlimited amount ✓ Osteoinductive, ✓ Osteoconductive ✓ Various mineral composition: cortical, cortico-cancellous, cancellous ✓ Various form: powder, cancellous cubes, cortical chips/fresh, fresh-frozen, freeze-dried/mineralized, demineralized	• No osteogenesis: no live-cell inclusion Disease transmission: viral or bacterial, 12.9–13.3% • High cost Dependent on donor's bone state: age Ethical problem
Xenograft	✓ No morbidity of donor site ✓ Unlimited amount ✓ Osteoconductive	• No osteogenesis • No osteoinduction • Disease transmission • Non-resorbable *In Vivo* • Ethical problem

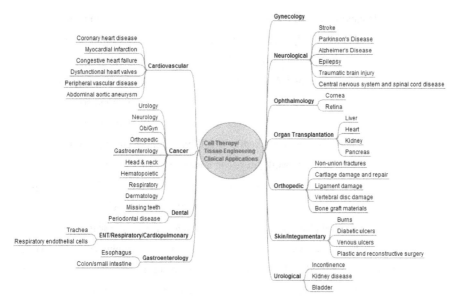

Figure 1.2 Application of Tissue Engineering and Regenerative Medicine (TERM)

(https://www.healthworkscollective.com/applications-global-markets-tissue-engineering-and-cell-therapy/)

The application of tissue engineering is found almost in all medical sciences, such as cardiovascular, dental, neurological, skin, orthopedic, etc. However, tissue engineering is still in infancies for many areas, and investigators are coming day by day with their new ideas and techniques for organ regenerations. The most acceptable application of tissue engineering has been found in orthopedics, with many more exploration opportunities. The first scientific literature on calcium phosphate-based ceramic biomaterial was reported in 1920 [8]. However, hydroxyapatite (HA) granules for bone defect repair were published in the early 1950s, and self-hardening calcium phosphate cement (CPC) was developed and reported in the late 1980s [9]. An extensive study on various parameters related to bone regeneration has been carried out after the 1980s. It includes the research associated with different biomaterials for their potential use as bone substitute material [10]–[17], finding the best suitable structure favorable for bone growth [18]–[25], Cell biomaterial interaction [26]–[28], and use of various growth factor for extracellular matrix (ECM) formulation [29], [30], and more importantly design the scaffold or construct for multi-parameter functionality [18], [31]–[36].

While looking toward BTE, we found that calcium phosphate group materials are highly prevalent and clinically accepted due to their similar mineral composition to that of bone. In this group, the HA, Beta phase of tricalcium phosphate (β-TCP), biphasic Calcium phosphate (BCP), (blends of HA and TCP) are comprehensively clinically established during the last 30 years [12], [37], [38]. The new class of ceramic materials, including zirconia, Alumina, magnesium oxide, etc., is considered to improve the engineered constructs' osteoinductive, osteoconductive, stability, and mechanical properties scaffold [39]–[42]. Many researchers work on a composite of some polymer biomaterial and ceramic for enhancing osteoinduction, cell attachment, and cell proliferation [43]–[45]. The results of the study are stirring towards the new era of tissue engineering.

Another field of research is on the fabrication techniques of a scaffold. It includes various methods like conventional technique and additive manufacturing (AM) to customize printed scaffolds [4]. Traditional fabrication consists of methods like solvent casting, particulate leaching, sol-gel techniques, freeze-drying, gas foaming, etc. [4]. This method's significant advantage is easy in fabrication, where poor mechanical reliability, poor connectivity of pores, and non-standard pore size are the disadvantages. Modern technological assessment tools like rapid prototyping (RP), referred to as 3D Printing, are popular nowadays to overcome these disadvantages. It not only provides freedom for multiple design variations, but suitable mechanical integrity can also be achieved. With additive manufacturing, it is possible to work on numerous biomaterials and live-cell printing called bio-printing.

The scaffold's primary role in tissue engineering is to provide temporary structure reliability until the body's Extracellular matrix (ECM) is generated. Several studies have been reported for this ECM formulation, including the use of bioactive molecules such as vascular endothelial growth factor (VEGF), fibroblast growth factor (FGF), epithelial growth factor (EGF), glycosaminoglycans (GAGs), accompanying mechanical stimulation, surface modification, and designing of engineered construction with control porosity for natural vascularization [15][46]. Such growth factors and stimulation not only result in ECM formulation but also helps in angiogenesis. Last decade the more concentration was towards multifunctionality of scaffold rather than only bone regeneration. The main objective is to design the scaffold to execute two or more functions like bone regeneration, drug delivery and growth factors, etc.

1.2 The genesis of the research and its novelty

The next generation of bone tissue engineering is about incorporating drug molecules or signaling molecules for effective treatment. There is always a conflict between the drug delivery routes. Ginebra et al. hypothecated diffusion mainly controlling the drug release from the cement matrix [47]. On the other hand, Downes et al. claimed that diffusion and biomaterial surface degradation is responsible for drug delivery [48]. From both the study, it is clear that the biomaterial can be used to release the drug at a controlled rate during treatment of bone infection termed called osteomyelitis, bone tuberculosis (TB) arthritis, or any other bone bacterial infectious diseases [4]. In the proposed thesis, we determine the multifunctionality of ceramic 3D printed scaffolds. It is achieved by incorporating the antibiotic drug to achieve an acceptable regional drug delivery and tissue regeneration. The novelty lies in a comparative study on the effect of conventional and microwave sintering in terms of mechanical strength and other derived properties for ceramic materials.

1.3 An overview of the present research

To meet the objectives, the report is systematized into seven chapters. A brief outline of each chapter is given below:

Chapter 1: Introduction

This chapter comprises necessary information about tissue engineering and its importance. Further, it also an insight into the different materials that are used for bone regeneration.

Chapter 2: Literature review

This chapter highlighted literature related to bone tissue engineering. This chapter aims to emphasize the various available techniques, methods, and applications to determine the specific objective of the study. The literature has been completed for biomaterials, fabrication methods, pros and cons of each technique, and various drug liberation and management.

Chapter 3: Geometric modeling and finite element analysis of 3D printable CAD designs

This chapter deals with the geometric modeling of scaffold based on extrusion-based 3D printing process parameters and simulation to find the best suitable combination of composite and lay down a pattern of scaffolds.

Chapter 4: 3D printing of ceramic biomaterials

This chapter throws light on printing parameters and experimental procedures for four composites. Selected Composites are Case I- βTCP: HA (80:20); Case II-βTCP: Al_2O_3 (90:10); Case III- βTCP: MgO (90:10); Case IV-βTCP: ZrO_2 (90:10). The composite configuration has been decided as per finite element analysis (FEA) result and literature supports. For ease in fabrication and looking towards the most practical aspect, the laydown pattern, i.e., architecture followed for all cases, is 0^0-90^0 orientation. The various analysis was performed on a scaffold and discussed.

Chapter 5: Critical analysis of the sintering of ceramic biomaterials

This chapter compares conventional and microwave sintering on mechanical, Phase assemblage, morphology, and compositional analysis, and cytocompatibility testing of β-TCP: HA. For conventional sintering, the three different temperature 1000,1100,1200 ^0C was selected by altering binder concentration. The best result of these was compared with microwave sintering at 1200 ^0C.

Chapter 6: Conclusion

This chapter presents the summary of results, recommendations in the direction of scaffold fabrication and post-processing for ceramic composite materials. It also discusses the specific contributions made in this research work and their limitations. Implications of the findings and general discussions on the area of research work are covered in this chapter.

Chapter 7: Future Scope

This chapter discusses the research's future directions. It highlights the work that needs attention to consider and limitations while conducting the present work.

CHAPTER 2: LITERATURE REVIEW

2.1 Introduction:

Degenerative bone diseases and fractures are known to affect millions of people worldwide [49]. The surgical treatment for bone diseases involved autograft (transplant within the same body), allograft (transplant within the same species), and Xenograft (transplant between different species). The first technique is considered the standard criterion in clinical practice, but it has some disadvantages like donor-site morbidity, the need for a second surgery, anatomical constraint, and hematoma formulation. Allograft has the problem of immunogenic rejection and disease transfer [6]. A xenograft is considered less expensive and abundant but has disadvantages of hyperacute or chronicle rejection, xerosis, and ethical issues.

The alternative way to employ regenerative techniques is often referred to tissue engineering for restoration, maintenance, and improving the tissue functions. The term' tissue engineering' was officially coined at a National Science Foundation workshop in 1988 [6] while Langer and Vacanti give the precise definition of tissue engineering in 1993 as "a multidisciplinary scientific branch that combines cell biology, regenerative medicine, materials science and engineering" [3], [4]. In recent years, the focus of bone tissue engineering (BTE) is towards the use of scaffold loaded with the sustained release of drug as a delivery system to heal the bone defect along with preventing recurrent infection will added value to BTE scaffolds [51], [54].

BTE consists of four components: angiogenesis, biomaterial, cell, and growth factor/drugs (Figure 1). Angiogenesis is about the formation of new blood vessels in the engineered tissue. In contrast, the biomaterial is used to fabricate a scaffold to provide temporary support to the cell and responsible for cell proliferation, differentiation, attachment, and extracellular matrix production for new bone formulation. The primary element of a living organism is a cell, and its functionality varies from organ to organ; every cell has a specific phenotype. For bone tissue engineering, two kinds of cells need to be considered: 1) Osteoblast 2) Osteoclast. The osteoblast cell is responsible for bone generation, whereas the osteoclast cell function is bone resorption [52]. Growth factor-like Bone Morphogenic Proteins (BMP), signaling molecules, drug (antibiotic, anti-inflammatory, antitubercular, etc.), and other supplements are responsible for cell differentiation and proliferation. Different possible drug administration routes are broadly classified into systematic, target base, and local drug delivery. The drug delivered systematically is absorbed into the bloodstream and distributed through the body's circulation system, resulting in systematic toxicity with liver complications and poor penetration into targeted tissue [53]. When the drug is delivered on a target base or locally, a systematic administration can be limited. A high amount of drug concentration can be reached to the target side. However, target-based drug delivery involves the use of ferromagnetic nanomaterials coated with a drug of interest, which can be moved to the magnetic field's target side and possess the disadvantage of again traveling through the body system, resulting in some drug dispensing and not that much effective when considering the patient with the metallic implant in a body. The drug delivered locally will be placed directly on the target side and found to be 200 times higher in concentration when compared with systematic drug administration [54].

Some of the prominent studies done on the multifunctionality of a scaffold. Bose et al. have demonstrated the use of bioceramic material for the drug, BMP proteins, and other vitamines delivery. They used 3D, a printed TCP scaffold, to control vitamin D_3 release to enhance healing due to enabling osteoblast proliferation[55], [56]. In another study, they employed controlled release of Soy Isoflavones for in vitro chemopreventive, bone-cell proliferating, and immune-modulatory potential [57]. Gbureck et al. have worked on the incorporation of a drug delivery system through a single-step low-temperature fabrication

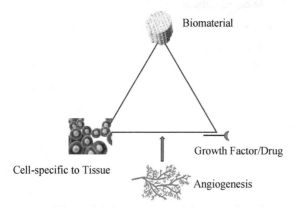

Figure 2.1 Components of tissue engineering

a process by using an inkjet printing process. They performed studies to find the correlation between drug release for the static and dynamic immersing conditions [58]. In another study, vancomycin release from 3D powder base printed scaffold is analyzed[59], [60]. Both the study gives the exciting results and act as inspiration for the multifunctionality of bioceramic materials. The current study will focus specifically on the rationale of scaffold fabrication techniques and their application to load different drugs relevant for treating pathologies associated with the bone repair process for osteomyelitis and bone tuberculosis, also called TB arthritis and other bone-related diseases.

2.2 Biomaterial:

In the first Consensus Conference of the European Society for Biomaterials (ESB) in 1976, a biomaterial was defined as "A nonviable material used in a medical device, intended to interact with biological systems." However, the ESB's current definition is "A material intended to interface with biological systems to evaluate, treat, augment or replace any tissue, organ or function of the body" [6]. Characteristically there are three individual groups of biomaterials: metal, ceramic, and polymer. Each group has its advantages concerning mechanical property, biocompatibility, and degradability. Butscher et al. reviewed the natural material with bulk biomaterial for mechanical properties (Figure 2). It gives insight into various biomaterials for their applications regarding Young's modulus and fracture toughness [61].

Variety of synthetic polymers like polystyrene, polylactic acid (PLA), polyglycolic acid (PGA), poly-dl-lactic-co- glycolic acid (PLGA), and Poly-l-lactic acid (PLLA), etc. possess advantages of controlled degradation, tailored architecture. However, they have a high degree of rejection due to reducing bioactivity and may cause necrosis [62]. The use of natural polymers such as collagen, various proteoglycans, alginate-based substrates, and chitosan retain benefits like bioactive, encouraging good cell growth and adhesion [63]. However, the fabrication of a homogenous and reproducible structure with superior mechanical property is a challenge.

The ceramic biomaterial's chemical and operational properties are similar to the mineral phase of natural bone. These materials are characterized by high mechanical stiffness (Young's modulus), hard, brittle surface, and low elasticity, making them more appropriate for bone regeneration. Hence the main focus of this thesis is on bio-ceramic material. However, the limitation of ceramic materials like brittleness, mimicking the real shape of implantation, challenging to control degradation rate, and unable to handle the mechanical load needed for remodeling limited its clinical evidence [6], [7–9].

The composition of tissues governs the engineered biomaterial matrix selection and design known as a scaffold. Ideally, an extracellular matrix (ECM) of bone comprises hydroxyapatite (HA) (biological ceramic) embedded with collagen matrix (biological polymer) and water. Each composition performs a specific function like biological ceramic accounts for approximately 70 % of the weight and provides compressive stiffness to the bone. While the organic matter: type I collagen gives the bone flexibility and elasticity, allowing it to stretch, bend, and twist. The key considerations to make while determining the scaffold for tissue engineering applications are listed in Table 2.1. In general, the tissue-engineered scaffold must have interconnected pores with a high amount of porosity, must be biocompatible and biodegradable along with mechanical reliability is anticipated. To promote angiogenesis, well-interconnected pores are highly desirable.

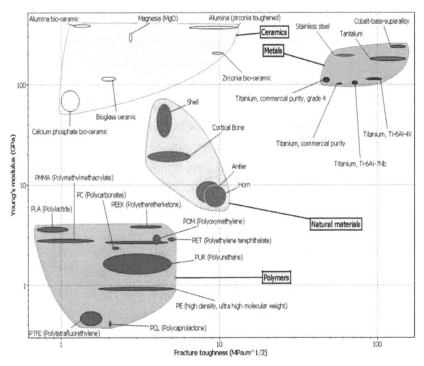

Figure 2.2 Mechanical properties of biomaterials along with bulk materials for a medical purpose [61]

Table 2.1 Features to be considered in scaffold biomaterial

Features	Ideal consideration or hypothesis	References
Biocompatibility	The cell's behavior with the biomaterial is such that it must adhere, function normally, and migrate onto a surface to proliferate before positioning the new matrix.	[1], [2], [50], [61], [12–20]
Osteoconductive	Encourage host bone for attachment and progress bone in growth into the scaffold	[50], [69], [73], [21–24],
Biodegradability	To permit replacing implanted scaffold or tissue-engineered construct by extracellular matrix generated by own body cells over the period.	[1-2], [50],[14], [15], [17], [18],[26],
Mechanical Property	The balance between mechanical properties and porosity of scaffold could result from cell infiltration and vascularization, which become the main criteria for any tissue-engineering construct's success.	[6], [69], [17], [18], [21], [27–33]
Scaffold architecture	The scaffold's structure representation with and interconnectivity and high porosity ensure cell penetration and adequate diffusion of nutrients. Additionally, it allows the dispersion of waste products out of the scaffold without the intervention of other organs and surrounding tissue.	[6],[52], [13–15], [17], [18], [24], [34–36],
Manufacturing technology	Developing accessible and affordable manufacturing processes with good manufacturing practice (GMP) standards is equally essential for the effective transformation of tissue engineering approaches to clinical practices.	[6], [14], [15], [17], [18], [37–41]
Commercialization	Fabricated at an acceptable cost for commercialization	[50], , [17], [18]

2.3 Scaffold fabrication techniques:

In tissue engineering, scaffolds provide temporary support to the structure and accommodate cell growth and tissue regeneration in a 3D matrix. Therefore, it is essential to consider the scaffold design parameters for bone tissue engineering. However, the configuration selection depends on the anatomical site of regeneration, the mechanical load on that site, and the desired rate of assimilation, like degradation rate. The necessary parameters are: first, high porosity and proper pore size with full interconnectivity for cell migration and nutrient delivery, second anatomical shape matrix with reproducibility, and rate of degradation that should be matched with healing rate, i.e., neither slow nor fast. Some other vital parameters are given by Temenoff et al. [36] and reviewed by B. Thavornyutikarn et al. [50] are listed in Table 2.2.

With the above parameters' cognizance, the various fabrication techniques evolved, broadly classified as conventional and non-conventional techniques. Each part is subdivided into the different processes explained graphically in Figure 2.3.

2.3.1 Conventional Scaffold fabrication techniques:

The brief of various available conventional techniques are as follows: B. Thavornyutikarn et al. studied the solvent casting process as the dissolution of the polymer-ceramic composite in an organic solvent and casting the solution into a predefined 3D mold. The solvent/porogen subsequently evaporates, leaving a scaffold behind [4-5],[15-16],[41],[43–47]. However, different porogen particles are added to control the scaffold's porosity and internal pore size [50], [46-47]. Freeze-drying also needs organic solvent or water, eliminating the use of any porogen particles. A synthetic polymer is dissolved in a suitable solvent and then poured into a predefined mold followed by lyophilization [50], [46-47]. Thermal-induced phase separation (TIPS) involves using an organic solvent to dissolve polymer mixed with or without ceramic. This polymer solution is rapidly cooled down, and the porous scaffold is obtained via sublimation [50],[93]. In gas foaming, a polymer is placed in the closed chamber and then saturated with high-pressure CO_2. As the pressure is instantly dropped, the thermodynamic instability results from nucleation and formation of pores [50],[93],[48–50]. To attain the ultimate interconnected network combination, particulate leaching and gas foaming was developed [50], [20]. In electrospinning, polymeric non-woven scaffolds are fabricated with the use of an electric charge. It possesses the advantage of scaffold fabrication with a wide range of fiber diameters from microns down to nanometer with good interconnectivity [50],[46],[51-52]. The powder foaming process is generally used to fabricate ceramic and glass scaffolds. A slurry of ceramic particles and glass is used to prepare the green body. Fillers such as sucrose, gelatin, PMMA microbeads, and wetting agent, i.e., surfactant, are added in suspension to produce porosity when burning during sintering [50],[93]. Sol-gel is an adaptable process involving condensation and gelation reaction to form a sol by adding surfactant. This technique is based on the chemical reaction of inorganic polymerization of metal alkoxides [50]. The particulars of each conventional process are given in Table 2.3.

Table 2.2 Scaffold design parameters for bone tissue engineering is given by Thavornyutikarn et al. [50]

Parameter	Requirement
Porosity	Maximum without compromising mechanical properties
Pore size	300-500 μm
Pore Structure	Significant for cell mobilization
Mechanical properties	Highly interconnected
Cancellous Bone	Tension and compression strength: 5-10MPa
	Modulus: 50-100 MPa
Cortical Bone	Tension Strength: 80-150 MPa
	Modulus: 17-20 GPa
	Compression strength :130-220 MPa
	Modulus: 17-20 GPa
	Fracture Toughness: 6-8 MPa$\sqrt{m}$
Derivative Properties	
Degradation Time	Must be tailored to match the application in patients
Degradation Mechanism	Bulk or surface erosion
Biocompatibility	No chronic inflammation
Serializability	Serializable without altering material properties

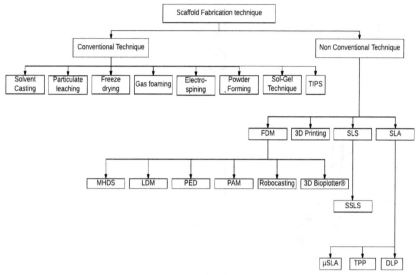

Figure 2.3 Various scaffold fabrication techniques

2.3.2 Limitations of the conventional process

Ideally, the tissue-engineering construct should be porous with suitable pore size and good interconnectivity to boost cell penetration, tissue ingrowth, and vascularization with nutrient delivery. It should provide good mechanical reliability and degradation rate matching the healing kinetics of injured bone [50]. The major limitation of conventional scaffold fabrication is the inability to address design/patient specificity. Although the conventional process owns its advantages, it cannot produce fully interconnected and uniform pore morphology in the scaffold. Additionally, pore geometry and pore size cannot precisely control with this technique and have poor reproducibility. Another limitation is that most conventional processes use an organic solvent, chemicals, and a porogen to produce pores, and their presence in a scaffold may cause inflammatory responses.

Table 2.3 Summary of conventional scaffold fabrication technique

Scaffold Fabrication process	Principle	Technique [94]	References
Solvent casting	Dissolve the polymer-ceramic composite in an organic solvent and cast the solution into a predefined 3D mold.		[4], [41], [43-47] [50]
Particulate leaching	In addition to the polymer solution, the porogen particle is being added to fabricate a porous scaffold. After the solvent evaporates, the dried scaffold is fractionated in water or a suitable solvent to remove particulate.		
Freeze drying	A synthetic polymer is dissolved in a suitable solvent and then poured in a predefined mold followed by lyophilization to produce a porous scaffold.		[4], [46], [47], [53]

Method	Description	Illustration	References
Thermal-induced phase separation (TIPS)	TIPS involves the use of an organic solvent to dissolve polymer mixed with or without ceramic. This solution is then rapidly cooled, followed by sublimation.		[50], [93]
Gas foaming/ Supercritical fluid processing	High-pressure gas is used as a porogen to create interconnected pores.		[46], [48–50]
Electrospinning	A polymeric non-woven scaffold is fabricated with the use of an electric charge.		[17], [46], [51], [52]
Powder foaming	A suspension of ceramic or glass slurry is used to prepare a green body, followed by sintering to burn our organic additive and build the porous structure.		[50], [93]
Sol-gel technique	Condensation and gelation reaction is used for forming a sol with the addition of surfactant.		[50], [93]

2.3.3 Non-conventional scaffold fabrication techniques

The conventional fabrication techniques were being tailored to fabricate scaffolds for specific tissue engineering applications and not generic. Each material or composite needs various processability to fulfill the scaffolds' requirements or tissue engineering construct. Among the critical requirement for scaffold fabrication, some important to be considered are: process condition, processability, repeatability, and consistency are still challenging in bone tissue engineering [25]. To attain this challenge, various solid freeform (SFF) techniques, also called Additive Manufacturing (AM) and Rapid Prototyping (RP), comes into existence. However, this term is ambiguous in two aspects. The focus is on freedom regarding geometry for manufacturability, not on speed, making the process slow when equated with conventional methods.

Furthermore, the technique implies a limited application for a pilot series, i.e., prototyping [61]. In essence, this technique is based on modern computer-aided design (CAD) and computer-aided manufacturing (CAM) tools. The complex structure is fabricated in a layer-by-layer routine, i.e., the addition of one layer over the other to builds via processing of powder, liquid, and solid sheets according to its digital cross-sectional 3D image.

The brief definition of technical terms used in SFF described in the user guide to rapid prototyping by Grimm et al. [99] is also listed alphabetically by Thavornyutikarn [50] (Please refer to the paper for more details). The technological flow chart of all SFF techniques is illustrated in Figure 2.4. The four most commonly used SFF techniques in tissue engineering are Stereolithography (SLA), Selective Laser Sintering (SLS), 3-Dimensional Printing (3DP), and Fused-Deposition-Modeling (FDM). These categories within the subgroup are mentioned in Figure 2.3

SFF offers many benefits, which are summarized as below [50],[25]:

1. Customized design: The sophisticated and nonlinear shape based on medical imaging techniques can fabricate with the instigation of CAD modeling.

2.Computer-controlled fabrication: The amalgamation of the computer into the manufacturing process leads to high accuracy, quality, and optimization in process parameters using minimum labor. This results in the fabrication of highly porous (up to 90 %) and the fully interconnected scaffold, making a remarkable effect on cell attachment, proliferation, and ECM formulation.

3. Anisotropic scaffold microstructures: The use of CAD-CAM and SFF approaches affects the anisotropic scaffold production, which has different mechanical properties at different zones of the same scaffold [50]. It helps in structuring multiple cell types as per necessity [55–59].

4. Processing conditions: SFF includes a solvent-free fabrication of the scaffold at room temperature, allowing the researcher to incorporate various body morphogenic proteins (BMP) and drugs during the scaffold fabrication [59-60]. Essentially SFF technique provides several advantages over the conventional fabrication concerning repeatability, consistency, accuracy, and precise control over the architecture and porosity of 3D printed scaffold, well summarized by Leong et al. It contributes towards the improvement in the performance of tissue construct regarding mechanical and biological properties [25], [50], [78], [102].

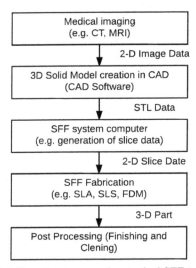

Figure 2.4 Flowchart presenting typical SFF technology

2.3.3.1 Stereolithography (SLA)

Chuck Hull introduced the first additive manufacturing process in 1986, known as 'Stereolithography (SLA). CAD data was guided to cure the printed monomer model (figure 2.5)[105]. The green body was fabricated as a result of the bonding of ceramic particles through curing. After curing each layer, the platform is lowered down for bottom-up fabrication, and a new layer of resin with ceramic practices spread on the surface. The polymer binder was removed by pyrolysis, and ceramic parts sintered to strengthen the part [16], [61-62]. Fisher et al. used SLA for the fabrication of poly (propylene fumarate) (PPF) 3D scaffold in the rabbit for cranial defect reconstruction [106]. The recent advancement in the material science library of resins with biodegradable moieties and cells' encapsulation during processing increases. Now SLA can be used to process a wide variety of materials like PCL, PDLLA, Poly (ester-anhydride), hydrogel polymer, poly (ethylene glycol), etc. are well-reviewed by Thavornyutikarn et al. [50].

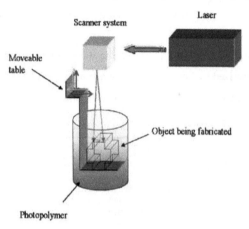

Figure 2.5 Stereolithography [105]

In 1996, Chu et al. attempted the use of SLA for scaffold fabrication using ceramic materials. Some researchers used the combination of SLA and investment casting for the indirect fabrication of bio-ceramic materials [106]. With the up-gradation of SLA technology of laser power, lateral and vertical resolution new generation of SLA has materialized. This new generation is micro-stereolithographic (µSLA), two-photon polymerization (TPP), and digital light processing (DLP) [50].

Later, µSLA has been developed to fabricate microstructure with precision. It involves using a single photon beam that focuses precisely on reducing the laser's spot size. Many researchers use µSLA for both polymers and ceramic scaffolds.

The advancement in the TPP system meant achieving a greater depth, high resolution at ultra-fast speed. While in DLP, dynamic masks are used to cure a whole layer, resulting in inconsiderably higher building speed [50].

2.3.3.2 Selective Laser Sintering (SLS)

The University of Texas developed the SLS technique in 1986 [50]. The CO_2 laser beam is used to sinter (or fuse) the target region of material powder lying on the powder bed, developing a scaffold layer. After solidifying the first layer, the bed is lower down by one-layer thickness, and the next layer of powder material is laid down on top of the bed by a roller [4], [6], [16], [37-38], [62] (Figure 2.6). In SLS, the loose powder act as a support structure, and the residual powder can be removed after the complete process. In SLS, the tissue construct is fabricated from any material such as metals, ceramic, and polymer available in powder. Fabrication of bioceramic scaffold has proven difficult, so the indirect method of coating ceramic powder with polymer and sintering is used. A novel technique of surface selective laser sintering (SSLS) has been developed to minimize heat transfer. It is different from the conventional about using laser power, laser intensity, and minimum volumetric shrinkage [50].

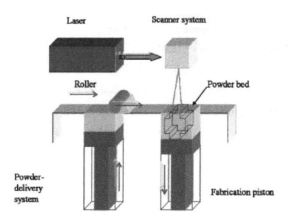

Figure 2.6 Selective Laser Sintering [105]

2.3.3.3 3D Printing (3DP)

3DP, a technology developed in the early 1990s at MIT, is a powder-based freeform fabrication method [71]. In 3DP solid is created by the reaction of liquid, which acts as a binder sprayed onto a powder bed [107]. The powder bed first performed the two functions as a reagent and second as physical support to the printed layer. This is an effortless and versatile technique used with any powder materials. The most common application is 3DP is for production of the ceramic scaffold and construct [50], [61], [71], [87], [89], [105], [108].

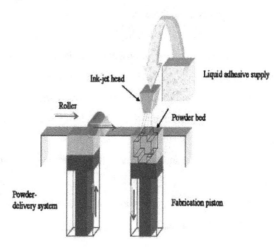

Figure 2.7 3D Printing [105]

2.3.3.4 Fused Deposition Modeling (FDM)

In FDM, the polymeric material is melted and extruded through the movable nozzle (normally in the X and Y axis) with a small orifice on the platform provided with z-direction movement [50]. In common with FDM, the process used two filament categories as model and support material. The support provided to the melted model layer can be detached either by breaking or solubilizing in some solvent liquid. After printing each layer as per CAD data, the platform is lowered in the Z direction for building another layer. Recently, with the improvement of FDM technology, a multi-nozzle system is being in practice. It gives the advantages of the printing of different materials with different properties to frame the optimum structure. [6], [16], [37-38], [62], [66-67].

FDM machines are explicitly developed for the home, school, small business with much lower price and less complexity than other SFF machines. Besides, low-cost reverse engineering and CAD freeware make the use of FDM gone viral [87]. However, the FDM process has been classified in another subcategory like Multi-head deposition system (MHDS), Low-temperature deposition manufacturing (LDM), precision extruding deposition (PED), pressure-assisted microsyringe (PAM), robocasting, and 3D-Bioplotter® system [50].

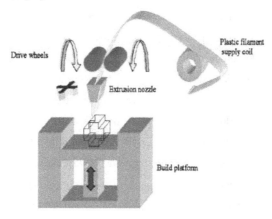

Figure 2.8 Fused Deposition Modeling [105]

2.4 Drug delivery using 3D printed scaffolds

It is anticipated that biodegradable scaffold material will degrade at the same rate of new bone formation. The slow degradation occurs a delay in developing new bone vascular growth, while fast degradation ensues in a partial filling of lesion area [69-70]. The next generation of bone tissue engineering is about incorporating drug molecules or signaling molecules for effective treatment. There is always a conflict between the drug delivery routes. Ginebra et al. hypothecated that the process of diffusion mainly controls the drug release from the cement matrix [47]. On the other hand, Downes et al. claimed that diffusion and biomaterial surface degradation is responsible for drug delivery [48]. From both the study, it is clear that the biomaterial can be used to release the drug at a controlled rate during treatment of bone infection termed called osteomyelitis, bone tuberculosis (TB) arthritis, or any other bone bacterial infectious diseases.

Two reasons cause osteomyelitis: 1) bacteremia spread to the bone causing infection 2) when the patient has an infection elsewhere in the body. Recent surgery and chronicle diseases like diabetes, HIV, Sickle cell, and open wound increase the chance of infection-causing osteomyelitis. The treatment consists of debridement of infected tissue followed by irrigation with an antiseptic solution and a 4-6 week of parenteral antibiotic treatment[113]. While TB arthritis is caused by a bacterium called mycobacterium tuberculosis and primarily affects the lung but can spread to other organs like the central nervous system leading to tuberculous meningitis; and the skeletal system causing infection of the joints, kidneys, and gastrointestinal systems. Poor parenteral antibiotic/ anti-tuberculosis penetration at an infected site is substantially avoided by high serum concentration for extended periods [73-74]. Increased drug doses given either intravenously or orally may result in adverse drug effects like nephrotoxicity, ototoxicity or can cause gastrointestinal side effects. One of the critical factors for successfully treating regional bacterial infections is effective drugs to reach the infected area [114]. It can achieve with effective local drug delivery and target-based drug delivery process. Both the system has the advantage of providing proper regional drug delivery and controlled release rate without risk of adverse drug reaction [74-75]. However, target base drug delivery is beyond the scope of this thesis.

Canale et al. did pharmacokinetics studies and showed that the local concentrations of antibiotics were 200 times higher than those achieved with systemic antibiotic administration [54]. The objective of using the drug carrier and bone regeneration can be club together and is more critical from this paper's aims. Usually, the drug-release kinetics follows Higuchi's law [115], at least at the initial stages (until the release of 60% drug is released) [47]. In the initial stage, the mass of drug liberated proportional to $\sqrt{t}$; in the second stage, the release of drug proportional to time followed; in the third stage, liberation is stabilized as the environment antibiotic concentration increases [47], [31]. The porosity and microstructure parameters play a significant part in the kinetics of drug release[47], [115], [116].

Various researchers worked on a variety of drug carrier agent like calcium phosphate cement (CPC)[47]; dicalcium phosphate dehydrates (DCPD), dicalcium phosphate (DCP)[76], hydroxyapatite (HA), monocalcium phosphate monohydrate (MCPM)[61], poly(lactic-co-glycolic acid) (PLGA), alpha-tricalcium phosphate (α-TCP), beta-tricalcium phosphate (β-TCP), tetra calcium phosphate (TTCP)[71]. However, still poly (methyl methacrylate) (PMMA) is a gold standard for drug delivery (explained in table 2.4). It may be due to two main reasons: PMMA is very readily available, and the company or doctors are not intended to use any other composite. Besides that, sound pieces of evidence for PMMA are available as compared with another drug carrier medium.

The development of a polymeric drug carrier vehicle like PMMA is not new and is used to reduce infection after surgery like a knee replacement, hip joint replacement, etc. The number of problems associated with this is: bone cement is not biodegradable and second surgery is needed to remove, 60-65 % of the drug remains trapped inside the beads which may results in nidus for infection, can create a physical barrier in new bone formation [117], the risk of recolonization of bacteria [118] and thermal effects during polymerization [119], [120].

To overcome this problem, a biodegradable drug carrier agent has been famous nowadays. As the biodegradable bead is degradable inside the body, it eliminates the need for second surgery required for its removal; the material can be tailored to adjust the drug release rate. As the carrier dissolved inside, it does not act as a barrier in a new bone generation. PMMA is best when considering the load-bearing part of the bone. In contrast, for none or little load-bearing area, biodegradable materials are superior concerning drug entrapped and liberated through it [121].

On the other hand, some shreds of evidence showed that the biofilm formation by the bacteria, such as Staphylococcus aureus and Staphylococcus epidermis, limits the activity of antibiotics [122]. This biofilm can adhere to non-degradable drug carriers like PMMA, making it highly unsuitable as a drug delivery vehicle [122]. As the biodegradable bead is degradable inside the body, it eliminates the need for second surgery required for its removal; the material can be tailored to adjust the drug release rate. As the carrier dissolved inside, it does not act as a barrier in a new bone generation.

Ethell et al. did a comparative study for drug release in CPC and PMMA. The result indicated a faster antibiotic release from CPC than polymer [123]. Otsuka et al. found during *In Vitro* study that drug liberation increases with porosity. It serves as a shred of evidence to conclude that the drug kinetic follow the modified Fick's law [32]. A variety of fabrication processes is used to produce drug-loaded scaffolds for bone tuberculosis, osteomyelitis, and any bone infection disease conditions [22-23], [72], [74], [94–104]. The most common is to have drug impregnation to form a mesoporous powder, followed by 3D printing. Kun Li et al. evaluated the use of mesoporous bioactive glass (MBG) as a drug vehicle due to its bioactive and drug release functionality. He did a comparative study between pure β TCP and MBG. He found that the drug release level is above the minimum inhibitory concentration [MIC] for more than 12 weeks to maintain effective local concentration in MBG [135].

β-TCP scaffold embedded with rifampicin and isoniazid in combination prevent the drug resistance in M. tuberculosis and provide a bactericidal effect along with a reduction in liver toxicity resulted due to high drug concentration [67]. Efforts made to use bio-ceramic and bio-composite as a drug carrier matrix. According to some researchers, the effect of drug addiction in ceramic increases injectability, mechanical strength (25 % in compression and 80 % inflection), which was attributed to decreased porosity and smaller precipitated crystals [47], [136]. However, some researchers had used polymer nanoparticle materials as a biodegradable drug carrier [137].

Wang et al. researched the use of PLA/PGA with cefazolin and gentamicin. They concluded that increasing the size of beads or adopting multilayer beads can increase the active release period of the drug [138]. Ueng et al. worked on prolonging antibiotic release by using poly-L-lysine coating, lyophilization, and increasing alginate content [77]. Ambrose et al. worked on the different formulation of polymeric drug carriers and found that 99 % PLGA-1 % tobramycin-0 % PEG would take approximately 186 days for all antibiotic release [113], [139]. He also achieves improvement in antibiotic Delivery by using microspheres in the animal model [113].

Stigter et al. assessed the use of tobramycin in biomimetic hydroxyapatite coating on titanium implants. Results opened the door to a new antibiotic delivery era to the surgical site after implantation to prevent post-surgical infections in orthopedics or trauma [134]. The table gives the details of different biomaterial uses as drug delivery agents and its advantage and disadvantages:

Table 2.4 Summary of various drug-carrying material

Materials	Drug	Advantage (+)/ Disadvantage(-)	Reference
PMMA (polymethylmethacrylate)	Vancomycin, Tobramycin or Gentamicin, Fosfomycin, Sodium Fusidate{46}	- Non-degradable, - The second surgery for bead removal is needed. - Act as a surface on which microbes adhere and grow on and potentially develop resistance to the antibiotic. - The heat generated due to the polymerization process results use of only heat resistive antibiotics. - Only a limited amount of antibiotic release from the total amount of antibiotic drugs embedded in PMMA.	[8], [22], [74], [88], [92], [96–98], [102], [110–114]

		- It also inhibits local immune response resulting from damaging phagocytic immune cells. + PMMA is a better carrier for sodium fusidate + Easily available at cheap rates. + Simple in fabrication at the bedside. + Variation in drug and its capacity can be adjusted as per need.	
Calcium sulfate	Moxifloxacin, Vancomycin	- Inflammatory reactions because of cytotoxic effects being observed. + Delivery of heat-sensitive antibiotics can be possible. + Moxifloxacin was found to be effective in treating Methicillin-resistant Staphylococcus aureus osteomyelitis with the lower bacterial load locally throughout the study period. + As it is fully absorbable, local antibiotics can be delivered without removing the beads.	[76], [127], [114], [115]
polylactic acid (PLA)		- Decreased bone regeneration due to acidic degradation material + Controlled degradation rate can be achieved with this drug delivery system.	[22], [102], [116], [117]
polycaprolactone (PCL)			
polylactide-polyglycolide copolymers (PLGA)	Penicillin, Tobramycin	+ Fairly steady antibiotic release. + Linear release of antibiotics can be obtained. + Biodegradable antibiotic beads may provide an extended bactericidal concentration of antibiotics for the time needed to complete the treatment.	[22], [74], [82], [109], [116], [117]

PLA/PGA (50:50)	Cefazolin, Gentamicin, Tobramycin	+ Increasing the size of the beads or adopting multi-layered beads, a sufficient drug release period can be increased.	[37], [113], [139]
NaCl	Vancomycin and gentamicin	+ Delivery of two different antibiotics can be achieved	[125]
poly-L-lysine-coated alginate beads	vancomycin	+ By increasing the alginate content in the technique of ploy-L-Lysine coating followed by lyophilization, the antibiotic release was prolonged.	[77]
HA composite (HA-PoP-CTS)	Vancomycin, Fosfomycin, Sodium Fusidate	+ Suitable carrier for vancomycin and fosfomycin	[132]
hydroxyapatite	Vancomycin	+ It does not require a second surgery for removal, making it the more attractive of the two options + HA is osteoconductive and helps in bone regeneration.	[133]
calcium phosphate (CaP) in combination with			
(CaP): silica	vancomycin, tobramycin	+ Overcome the limitations of PMMA delivery systems and stimulate the new bone restoration	[76]
(CaP): (b-TCP), (DCP)	tobramycin	+ Expected to combat infection and eliminate the dead space along with stimulating bone regeneration.	[76]
(CaP):b-TCP–PLA nanocomposites	vancomycin	+ Slowly release antibiotic with potent antimicrobial activity can be achieved.	[76]

(CaP):b-TCP–PCL (CaP): DCP–PCL	vancomycin, tobramycin	+ Eliminate the need for removal surgery and promote repairing the osseous defect with tissue engineering strategy.	[76]
(CaP): Alginate (CaP): Chitosan	tobramycin	+ Retard in drug liberation.	[126], [148]
polyacrylic acid (PAA)	gentamicin	+ Drug delivery for an extended period is possible with the use of PAA of high molecular weight.	[47], [126]

2.5 Discussion

The problems associated with the implants are a mismatch of mechanical properties between the implant and surrounding tissues, which can lead to stress shielding near the periphery of the implant and consequently inhibit tissue growth or cause implant loosening [68], [149], [150]. This encourages bio-engineers to start striving for cell base and tissue engineering bone regeneration. The scaffold's role in BTE is to provide mechanical support for bone ingrowth within the surrounding tissues. However, the single ceramic biomaterial cannot solve this purpose, as each of them has its benefit and detriment. Hence, the composite scaffold providing a combined advantage with optimization in slurry's rheological properties is critical. Kalita et al. conveyed the fabrication of PP (polypropylene) – TCP scaffold using the FDM approach [151]. Liu et al. worked on silica- Hydroxyapatite, titanium, and silica scaffold fabricated from SLS followed by sintering at 1200^0C and 900^0C in particular cases and reported improvements in compressive strength was achieved [151], [152]. Sapkal et al. work extensively on the use of the HA-TCP composite scaffold for controlled degradation, while in another study, he worked on HA-ZrO_2 for improving the strength of scaffold using indirect fabrication technique [39], [75].

Yuan showed by MTT and toxicity result that composite material has excellent tissue compatibility, loading efficiency and did not impact drugs *In Vivo* [67]. Butscher et al. reviewed different material approaches, including polymer, ceramic, and composite, based on particle size and binder for bone tissue engineering [61]. Mart et al. studied the use of gelatin and silicon-doped hydroxyapatite (HASi) for an ideal synthetic composite scaffold material. The group tried to optimize the rapid prototyping of drug-loaded composite scaffolds to work in mild conditions. He reported that the scaffold's compressive behaviour is similar to that of trabecular bone for the same density with the benefit of gelatin involving biological property like cell differentiation, gene expression, and drug release profile matching the Noyes-Whitney equation [70].

On the other hand, some cases have reported improved mechanical properties by using inorganic compounds such as calcium phosphates and silicate bioactive glasses with biodegradable polymers. The degradability of such an inorganic compound increases drug elution time compared with pure ceramic [70], [153]. Bioactive glass is renowned as a Class A bioactive material [53] due to its contribution to osteoconduction and osteoproduction. This gives rise to bioglass composition with polymers, but the problem with this material is high brittleness and low fracture toughness [50]. Cao and Ku-boyama testified PGA/B-TCP composite and evaluated enhancement in new bone formation and osteoconductivity in rat femoral epicondyles compared with PGA/HA and Implant accessible controls [92]. Li et al. demonstrated the use of anti-TB drugs isoniazid (INH) and rifampicin (RFP) into the composite scaffold made up of mesoporous bioactive glass (MBG) and poly (3- hydroxybutyrate-co-3-hydroxyhexanoate) has excellent potential for the treatment of osteoarticular TB [135]. The development of the composite drug delivery system alone is extensive research, and numerous new findings came out on day today. Makarov et al. combined the calcium phosphate ceramic and degradable polymer and found the drug elution depends on composite porosity and homogeneity [76]. In one more study, Buranapanitkit et al. studied the efficacy of ceramic composite material with an antibiotic against the treatment of Methicillin-Resistant Staphylococcus Aureus (MRSA). He found the biodegradable composite an excellent carrier for vancomycin and fosfomycin, which was used as an anti-treatment drug for MRSA [132].

While searching for the *In Vivo* study, we found many studies use calcium phosphates like HA and TCP due to their chemical and structural similarity to the mineral phase of bone[92], [154]. However, these materials have poor mechanical properties while comparing with those of human bone. The compressive strength of calcium phosphate material is very high. Still, it has low tensile and fracture toughness, which restricts its application to the non-load bearing area even though its excellent biocompatibility and osteoconductivity [50].

A successful scaffold for bone regeneration depends on various parameters like biocompatibility, degradation rate, strength, cell proliferation rate, and, most importantly, its ability to help in angiogenesis. Lack of angiogenesis or vascularization in scaffolds is a crucial challenge, and improving blood vessel formulation strategies is one of the areas requiring the greatest extensive research. [2], [11], [126-127]. Consequently, the next generation of researchers is trying to emerge the next level of research with more sophisticated biomimetic material and integrated multifunctionality [155], [157].

2.6 Research objective

Based on exhaustive Literature review on almost all topic related to bone tissue engineering following objectives has been decided:

- Finite element analyses of 3D printable CAD designs for ceramic composite scaffolds achieve optimal strength, porosity, and composite concentration. It helps to understand the final scaffold behavior in terms of mechanical strength and acts as a decision-making tool for further experimentation.
- Develop a methodology for 3D printing using extrusion base printers with material βTCP, HA, Al_2O_3, MgO, and ZrO_2. Every composition needs different printing conditions and results in different mechanical and biological properties.
- To incorporate drugs in fabricated scaffold and prove a scaffold's multifunctionality, especially in bone infection disease treatments.
- To perform a critical analysis of conventional and microwave sintering parameters for ceramic materials suitable for tissue engineering application.

CHAPTER 3: GEOMETRIC MODELING AND FINITE ELEMENT ANALYSIS OF 3D PRINTABLE CAD DESIGNS OF SCAFFOLD

3.1 Introduction

Significant bone defects caused by trauma, accidents, or medical conditions can be treated by prosthetic implants, autograft, or allograft bone tissue. Nevertheless, there are some limitations like patient pain, immune reaction, disease transmission, and non-optimal interaction between the body and implanted materials. Bone tissue engineering (BTE) provides a promising solution to the above problems by producing a functional substitute for damaged tissue. Langer et al. defined tissue engineering as "a multidisciplinary scientific branch that combines cell biology, regenerative medicine, materials science and engineering" [4], [7].

The two significant tissue engineering components are cells: The primary components of a living organism, and the biomaterials: used for fabricating the scaffold functioning as a provisional mechanical support and responsible for cell migration, proliferation, differentiation [4]. A variety of metal, polymer, and ceramic biomaterials are being employed for BTE and reviewed by many authors [6], [61], [158]–[160]. Out of available biomaterials, the mineral phase of natural bone is similar to that of ceramic biomaterials described by mechanical stiffness (Young's modulus), hard, brittle surface, and low elasticity established it as appropriate for bone regeneration [4], [17], [161]. Hydroxyapatite (HA), β Tricalcium Phosphate (β-TCP), Magnesium (Mg), Silicate, Alumina (Al_2O_3), and zirconia (ZrO_2) are the most common material used in tissue engineering. Sapkal et al. works on HA–β-TCP [75]; β-TCP-Zirconia [40]; β-TCP [85] and found the improvement in mechanical strength with the addition of HA, zirconia while comparing with β-TCP in several papers. Mart et al. studied the Si-doped HA with gelatin for producing the micro and macropores in the scaffold for effective drug delivery and bone regeneration[70]. Si-doped HA is used for bone regeneration with promising results, and osteoinduction is shown by Vila et al. [162]. These are the few studies to represent the improvement in biomechanical properties of the scaffold.

The perfect scaffold for BTE must have the highest interconnectivity, high porosity, biocompatible, and biodegradable, along with mechanical reliability is expected. However, modern scientific techniques have produced a wide range of composite materials with osteoconductive and osteoinductive properties. Nevertheless, porosity and interconnectivity mainly depend on the scaffold fabrication process employed. The review paper by the same author described the various scaffold fabrication processes with their advantages and disadvantages [4]. The paper concludes the benefits of 3D printing over other conventional fabrication in terms of customized design, Computer control fabrication, anisotropic scaffold fabrication, and processing conditions [4], [50], [88], [163]–[168]. A current challenge in the 3D printing process is balancing mechanical property, porosity, interconnectivity, and pore size. It is impossible to fabricate the scaffold and test for the desired parameters as 3D printing is slow, time-consuming, high energy consumption, and expensive. The computer simulation provides an alternative tool for predicting mechanical property concerning the different scaffold design parameters. It saves time and helps the researcher know more about the scaffold's mechanical behavior *in Vivo* by simulation. The present article deals with the finite element simulation for predicting the effective modulus for different bio-ceramic composites to match the cortical bone characteristics.

3.2 Materials

Calcium phosphate-based materials are universally accepted in BTE applications because of their structural and chemical similitude to bone mineral and their natural features for osteoconductivity, osteoinductivity, cell attachment, cell proliferation, etc. desired for bone tissue regeneration[75]. The primary ceramic material used in tissue engineering is β-Tricalcium phosphate {β-TCP} ($Ca_3(PO_4)_2$), Zirconium (ZrO_2), Magnesia (MgO), Alumina (Al_2O_3), Hydroxyapatite {HA} ($Ca_{10}(PO_4)_6(OH)_2$). Although β-TCP is an auspicious bone replacement material that can construct a direct chemical bond with tissue week mechanical strength, rapid resorption restricted its practices [23], [169]. ZrO_2 is capable of promoting cell proliferation, differentiation in osteogenic conduit with Superior mechanical properties and biological features such as low corrosion potential, low cytotoxicity with minimal adhesion of bacteria [40], [42], [170], [171]. MgO has excellent biocompatibility, nontoxic with a reasonable rate of bone formation, and required biomechanical properties, making it suitable for tissue engineering application [172]–[174]. Al_2O_3 takes high hardness, low friction coefficient, excellent corrosion resistance, meager wear rate, inhibiting static fatigue, and slow crack growth while under load, making it competent for hard tissue replacement [170]. HA is one of the main mineral components of bones and teeth with excellent biocompatibility with skin and mussels tissues and unique physio-mechanical properties[171].

Determining the best material or composite for bone regeneration is a difficult task. Therefore, researchers work on different thoughts and aim to improve particular biomechanical properties crucial from their perspective. Out of all essential features, the scaffold's primary aim is to work as an extracellular matrix for cell growth and provide mechanical strength to the lesion area. The present study aims to identify the effect of scaffold architecture design from mechanical aspects. The study is divided into three parts:

1. To study the impact of architecture design on the porosity of the scaffold.
2. Finite element analysis of scaffold with altered design parameters for mechanical strength
3. Relationship between porosity and effective Young's modulus for optimum design architecture among the proposed one.

The mechanical properties considered in the present study are explained in Table 3.1

Table 3.1 Biomaterials and their properties

Materials	Mechanical Property		Ref.
	Young's Modulus (E)- GPA	Poisson's ratio (μ)	
β-Tricalcium phosphate (β-TCP), $(Ca_3(PO_4)_2)$	120	0.3	[12]
Zirconium (ZrO_2)	210	0.31	[42]
Magnesia (MgO)	300	0.35	[172]
Alumina (Al_2O_3)	320	0.23	[170]
Hydroxyapatite $(Ca_{10}(PO_4)_6(OH)_2)$	13	0.27	[171]

3.2.1 Composite material properties

The ceramic material alone cannot hold all the properties needed by an ideal scaffold and hence needs to build composite with other materials to account for the characteristic of interest. Tarafder et al. demonstrate that the MgO dopant TCP scaffold results in a 37 to 41% improvement in mechanical strength and improved osteogenesis during *In Vivo* Study in the Rabbit model [175]. Aminzare et al. found an increase in hardness from 2.52 to 5.12 GPa and 40 % enhancement in bending strength of scaffold by using alumina when reinforced with HA due to the formation of calcium aluminates [176]. Matsumoto et al. reported that when the mixing ratio of ZrO_2/HA is 70/30, the scaffold's strength is equal to cortical bone and high osteoconductivity during in-vivo experiments [42]. Sapkal et al. initiate TCP/ZrO₂ in the ratio of 70/30 to get the best suitable property for tissue engineering construct with indirect casting and 3D printing process [40] [39]. In another study by Sapkal et al., he found that TCP/HA ratio 80/20 will give the best result from different mixing ratios in biomechanical stability [75].

The mechanical properties of powder composite are difficult to calculate due to molecular changes at sintering. Nevertheless, the modified rule of the mixture, also known as the Halpin-Tsai Equation, can give accurate values [177] [178].

$$E_c = \frac{E_m(1 + 2s \times q \times V_p)}{(1 - q \times V_p)}$$

Where
$$q = \frac{(\frac{E_p}{E_m} - 1)}{(\frac{E_p}{E_m} + 2s)}$$

The formula can calculate Poisson's ratio of the composite:

$$\mu_c = \frac{\mu_m(1 + 2s \times q \times V_p)}{(1 - q \times V_p)}$$

Where
$$q = \frac{(\frac{\mu_p}{\mu_m} - 1)}{(\frac{\mu_p}{\mu_m} + 2s)}$$

Where E_c, μ_c are Young's modulus and Poisson's ratio of composite; E_m, μ_m are matrix Young's modulus and Poisson's ratio of material and E_p, μ_p Young's modulus and Poisson's Ratio of particle reinforced material, V_p The volume fraction of particle reinforced, and S is particle aspect ratio considered one as particle morphology is considered spherical. Accordingly, the modified Young's modulus and Poisson's ratio for various composites used in the proposed FEA are explained in Table 3.2

Table 3.2 Young's modulus and Poisson's ratio of matrix (β-TCP) material with other particle reinforced; where Ec (MPa) & μC are Young's modulus and Poisson's ratio of composite

Particle reinforced in a composite.	Composite proportion									
	90:10		80:20		70:30		60:40		50:50	
	E_c	μ_c	E_c	μ_c	E_c	μ_c	E_c	μ_c	E_c	μ_c
Zirconium (ZrO₂)	127.341	0.301	135.000	0.302	142.973	0.303	151.311	0.304	160.000	0.305

Magnesium (Mg)	132.412	0.304	145.722	0.309	159.991	0.314	175.351	0.319	191.991	0.324
Alumina (Al_2O_3)	133.332	0.293	147.681	0.286	163.195	0.278	179.992	0.272	198.242	0.264
Hydroxyapatite ($Ca_{10}(PO_4)_6(OH)_2$)	105.393	0.297	91.921	0.294	79.472	0.291	67.911	0.288	37.164	0.285

3.3 Methodology:
3.3.1 Geometrical modeling of the scaffold

Scaffolds were designed based on models suggested by Chuan et al. [179] while keeping in mind the extrusion-based 3D printing principles. The main parameters for scaffold design are strand diameter (D), pore diameter (d), and the orientation angle (θ) of the plotted layer concerning the previous layer. This parameter is responsible for scaffold architecture design. The scaffold architecture was noted as D_d_θ and denoted in Figure 3.1. Strand diameter (D) was selected based on needle size commercially available for extrusion-based 3D printing along with supportive evidence of previous literature and was taken as 400,600, 800 μm [40] [75] [180].

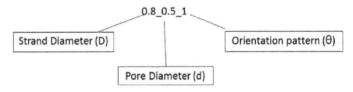

Figure 3.1 The nomenclature used for scaffold architecture design

Ideally, any scaffold consists of two kinds of porosity first: micro-porosity where pore diameter(d) <50 μm responsible for initial cell adhesion, and secondly macro-porosity, where pore diameter is in between 50-1000 μm responsible for oxygen, nutrient delivery, and angiogenesis. The generation of micro-pores is not in control during the 3D printing process. It is an effect of evaporation of binder particles between the two matrix particles unless some porogen is mainly used to create the micro-pores. The impact of these micro-pores on the mechanical aspect is considered negligible and not considered during the FEA. The macropores directly affect the mechanical strength of the scaffold and need to analyze for their effect. The ideal macro-pores size is still a matter of debate, but pores in the range of 300-500 μm are considered as favorable for nutrient delivery and blood vessel formation[50][68][181]. Therefore, in the present study, the pore diameter (d) 300, 400, and 500μm are considered. The orientation angle (θ) is the angle between two subsequent layers and responsible for the scaffold's different intricate architecture. The four different architecture decided for the present study and represented by number as in Table 3.3. By varying these three aspects of geometrical scaffold modeling, the total 36 scaffolds were designed in Computer-aided design software CATIA V5R20 (Dassault Système®), and analyses were done in ANSYS Workbench 16.2.

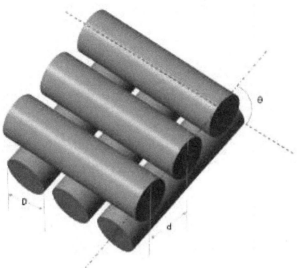

Figure 3.2

Architecture design parameters for scaffold

Table 3.3 Orientation angle representation

Sr no.	Layer orientation pattern
1	0-90
2	0-45-90-135
3	0-60-120
4	0-30-60-90-120-150

Table 3.4 An example of architecture design

(four orientation angles; three pore diameter and three-strand diameter lead to 36 design of scaffold was studied)

Architecture	3D view	Front view
0.4-0.5-1		
0.4-0.5-2		
0.4-0.5-3		
0.4-0.5-4		

3.3.2 Finite Element Analysis (FEA)

With the improvement in the computation facility, it is possible to predict material behavior and perform the simulation. Many efforts have been taken towards predicting the scaffold properties starting from cell structure (Simple Cubic (SC), Gibson Ashby (GA), Body-Centered Cubic (BCC), and Reinforced body-centred Cubic (RBCC).) by Luxner et al. [182] to using complicated Voronoi tessellation mathematical method for getting the bone-like structure and analyze it for cell penetration, nutrient diffusion and osteoconductive properties implemented by Gómez et al. [183]. Singh et al. performed the finite element simulation for comparing the compressive strength of stainless steel and Titanium alloy with compact bone by using the hollow cube unit cell suitable for SLS printing [184]. This method gives a close result but suitable only for scaffold produce with a hallow cube as a lattice structure and cannot be applied to another printing process, especially extrusion-based printing. Cahill et al. focused on accurate prediction of finite element prediction by improving the FEA modeling method, taking into account discrepancies like surface roughness and micro-pores. He concludes that ignoring these discrepancies leads to incorrect prediction [185]. The result of this work helps authors to have accurate modeling of the scaffold in the present study. Eshraghi et al. did a micro-mechanical investigation for polycaprolactone (PCL) and hydroxyapatite (HA) scaffold fabricated by SLS and found the FEA result in tune with the experimental method [186]. In another study by the same author, 1D, 2d, and 3D orthogonally, a porous scaffold was tested and analyzed by FEA. In both, the study fabrication process considered is SLS [187]. However, the author's best knowledge of FEA for the extrusion-based printing process with different architecture designs has not been found. Hence, it instigates the authors to work on the objective specified above.

Steps followed for FEA analysis are explained by Singhet al. [184] using Ansys workbench 16.2 and summarized as importing the CAD input file into FEA software as engineering data and assigning the composite material property followed by meshing with an element size of 300 μm. For analysis bottom of the model is constrained by fixed support at the bottom end, and displacement (0.001 mm, 0.002 mm, 0.003 mm, 0.004 mm) was applied at the top in a downward direction (Figure 3.3). For case study 1, Equivalent stresses (Von-Mises stresses) were noted, and for a case study, two reaction forces at the support were noted.

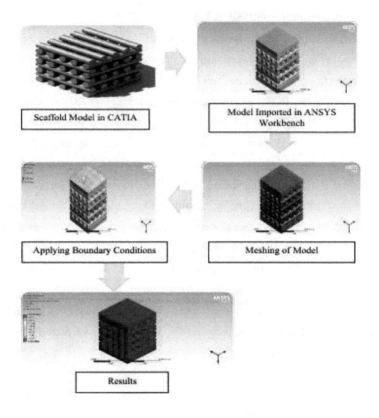

Figure 3.3 Schematic of steps of finite element analysis

3.4. Results and discussion

The FEA results for various architecture and composition was done and explained as below:

3.4.1 Porosity achieved with different architecture design

The porosity of a scaffold is the void space in the solid. The higher the porosity, the more space is available in the scaffold to form new tissue [188]. The porosity should preferably as high as possible. The porosity can be measured by the formula given below [189].

$$Porosity = 1 - \frac{V_{solid}}{V_{total}} \times 100\%$$

Where V_{solid}= Volume of Solid

V_{total} = Total Volume of Scaffold

The porosity values were 39.58 % to 64.13 %, depending on scaffold architecture and design. The average porosity is found out to be 51.63 %. The porosity found to be directly proportioned to design parameters strand diameter, pore diameter, orientation angle (Figure3.4)

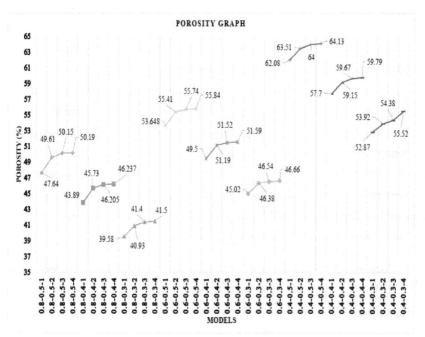

Figure 3. 4 Porosity of concerning architecture design of scaffold

Results show that strand diameter and pore diameter have a significant influence on the porosity of the structure. The larger the pore, the gap between the two strands; hence, void space will also be enormous; thus, porosity will increase with pore diameter, as shown in the results (Figure 3.4). On the contrary, the strand diameter has a negative response to porosity. Increasing strand diameter decreases the void space in the scaffold structure and reduces the scaffold's porosity.

The orientation angle (θ) also affects the porosity of the scaffold. The more intricate orientation higher the porosity, as represented in figure 3.4. The change in porosity is due to a change in surface area to volume ratio.

3.4.2 Case II Effect or architecture design and material composition on mechanical property

The Von-Mises stresses for four situations represented as S_1, S_2, S_3, and S_4 for β-TCP: ZrO_2, β-TCP: MgO, β-TCP: Al_2O_3 and β-TCP: HA respectively was analyzed. From pure matrix β-TCP (100:0), a 10 % increment in particle reinforced until 50 % was done. Figure 3.5 shows that Von-Mises stresses as a function of displacements for different concentrations of particles in the matrix. The mechanical property of composite depends on the mechanical property of components. ZrO_2, MgO, and Al_2O_3 possess superior mechanical properties than matrix material resulting in the higher percentage of this particle in the matrix will ultimately improve the mechanical property of composite. Therefore, the 50:50 ratio of matrix and particle material will show higher Von-Mises stress and eventually high compressive strength. However, ZrO_2 and Al_2O_3 material are not biodegradable, limiting their utilization in BTE. From FEA, it is recommended to have a small portion of around 10 %. However, MgO is the only material that possesses corrosion property when coming in contact with body fluid. This corrosion property restricted its utilization, and hence, the concentration should need to keep below 10 % HA has inferior mechanical properties than β-TCP, as represented in table 1.

Consequently, the mechanical properties of the composite should be lesser than pure β-TCP. Thus, HA shows the opposite trend as that of the first three materials. Nevertheless, β-TCP: HA will control the degradation rate of matrix material and helps in most-conduction, so recommended having in this composition between 20-30 %. In the present study, the particle's increment was considered 10 %, but to get more close and precise result, one should follow the FEA for a slight increase.

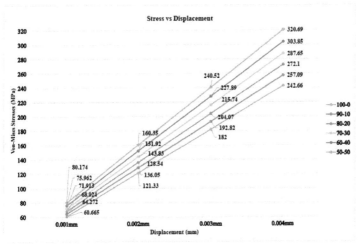

S_1

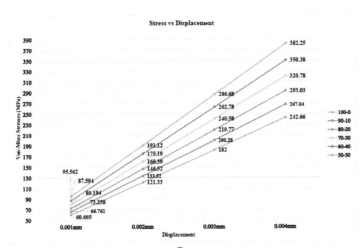

S_2

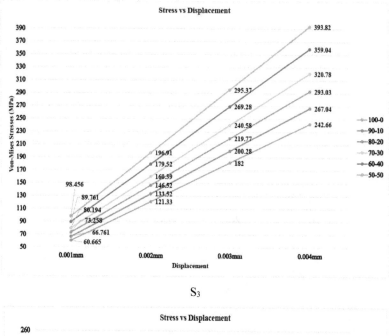

S₃

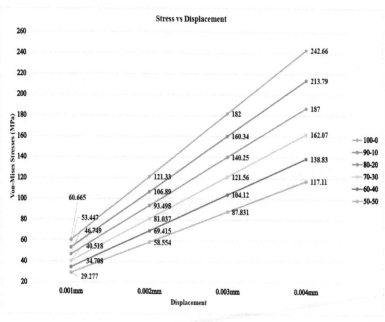

S₄

Figure 3.5 Von Mises stress for different composition: S_1, S_2, S_3, and S_4 for β-TCP: ZrO_2, β-TCP: MgO, β-TCP: Al_2O_3 and β-TCP: HA, respectively.

3.4.3 Relationship between Young's Modulus and Porosity of scaffold

The addition of Zirconia, Alumina, Magnesia in the composite will increase β-TCP's strength, sometimes more than the strength of bone, resulting in stress shielding. This can be avoided by calculating the effective modulus of the scaffold by below formula

$$E_{effective} = \frac{\frac{R}{A}}{\frac{dl}{l}}$$

Where R = Reaction forces at the fixed support; A = Cross Section Area; $\frac{dl}{l}$ = Axial Strain

The reaction force for each sample situation was calculated and represented in Figure.3.6. For S_1, the highest effective Young's modulus 28 GPa is shown by model 0.8_0.3_1 (Porosity 39.58%), and 0.4_0.5_4 (Porosity 64.13 %) has the lowest effective Young's modulus 2.2 GPa. While for S_2, the highest effective Young's modulus 33.2 GPa is shown by model 0.8_0.3_1 (porosity 39.58%), and 0.4_0.5_4 (porosity 64.13 %) has the lowest effective Young's modulus 4.1 GPa. For S_3, the highest effective Young's modulus 37.2 GPa is shown by model 0.8_0.3_1 (Porosity 39.58%), and 0.4_0.5_4 (Porosity 64.13 %) has the lowest effective Young's modulus 9.9 GPa. Whereas for S_4, the highest effective Young's modulus 19.5 GPa is shown by model 0.8_0.3_1 (porosity 39.58%), and 0.4_0.5_4 (porosity 64.13 %) has the lowest effective Young's modulus 0.8 GPa. The analysis revealed that the higher effective Young's modulus is associated with the largest strand diameter (D), smallest pores diameter (d), and highest orientation angle(θ), and vice versa for the lowest influential Young's modulus. It shows that effective young's modulus and porosity are inversely proportional to each other, while porosity is directly proportional to pore diameter and orientation angle. Figures 3.6 show the graphs of Effective Young's Modulus of scaffolds as a function of porosity. All the graphs follow the same trend showing declination in effective Young's modulus as an increase in porosity. Higher strand diameter and lower pore diameter in scaffold models show more effective Young's modulus as there is less gap between two strands providing more area at any cross-section of the scaffold. This makes a scaffold more stable for high compressive loads. As the strand diameter decreases and pore diameter increases (meaning the rise in porosity), the cross-section area drops, weakening the scaffold and hence declining its effective Young's modulus.

Considering Young's modulus of bone as 18.6 GPa. The optimum porosity and Young's modulus for S1: 0.6_0.5_2, for S2: 0.4_0.4_3 and for S3: 0.4_0.5_2 is found. While in S_4, the three-architecture design can be considered as optimum, that is 0.6_0.3_2; 0.8_0.4_4, and 0.6_0.3_3 showing clearly the adaptability of β-TCP: HA in many ways for tissue engineering application.

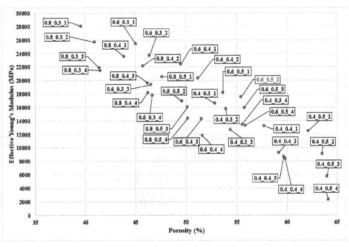

S_1

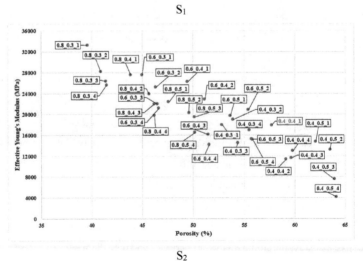

S_2

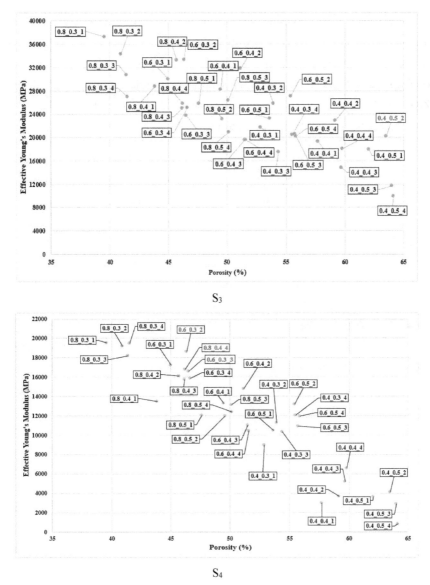

Figure 3.6 Effective Young's modulus Vs. Porosity graph for different composition: S_1, S_2, S_3, and S_4 for β-TCP: ZrO_2, β-TCP: MgO, β-TCP: Al_2O_3 and β-TCP: HA respectively.

3.5. Conclusion

The scaffolds were designed based on strand diameter, pore diameter, and orientation angle. A total of 36 scaffolds were intended on the combinations of properties for scaffolds. Each scaffold's porosities were determined and found that the strand and pore diameter significantly affected the scaffold's porosity. Before finding the optimum architecture design via FEA, it is necessary to find the compressive strength for various combinations of the composite. Accordingly, β-TCP is considered matrix material, and ZrO_2, MgO, Al_2O_3, and HA were analyzed with different concentrations. FEA has performed on this composite, and the following conclusion has been drawn:

1. for β-TCP: ZrO_2, the composite ratio of 90:10 will be promoted as an ideal combination by looking towards its non-degradability with the architecture of 0.6_0.5_2 of a balance between porosity and effective young's modulus matching towards the natural bone.
2. For β-TCP: MgO, the composite ratio of 90:10 and the architecture of 0.4_0.4_1 gives the desired scaffold properties closely matching with the cortical bone.
3. For β-TCP: Al_2O_3, the composite ratio 90:10 and architecture 0.4_0.5_2 provide higher porosity and excellent mechanical stability required for BTE.
4. For β-TCP: HA, the composite ratio of 80:20 or 70:30 with 0.6_0.3_2, 0.8_0.4_4, and 0.6_0.3_3 can provide the best combination of porosity and effective young's modulus close towards the bone tissue.
5. The result of porosity and young modulus comparison for all architectural designs will help decide the optimum plan for a scaffold in BTE.
6. The FEA simulation will reduce the number of trials and time to determine the optimum scaffold architecture to be used.

CHAPTER 4: 3D PRINTING OF CERAMIC BIOMATERIALS

4.1 Introduction

The design without manufacturing constrain is only possible to achieve with the help of 3D printing. 3D printing is associated with many advantages in bone tissue engineering like customization in design, minimum human intervention, anisotropic scaffold microstructures, the verity of processing condition, incorporation of live cells and bone morphogenetic proteins (BMP) during the printing process [25], [50], [97], [98], [100]–[102]. A prodigious effort has been put towards using all different additive manufacturing in tissue engineering. It includes the use of Fused deposition modeling (FDM) techniques for producing first generation of scaffolds [103], and move towards another advance additive manufacturing techniques like Multi-head deposition system (MHDS) [43] ,[190], [191], Low-temperature deposition manufacturing (LDM) [192] [193], precision extruding deposition (PED) [194] [195] [196], pressure-assisted microsyringe (PAM) [30], [197], robocasting [29], [193], and 3D-Bioplotter® system [4], [199]–[203]. Most of the rapid prototyping systems are allowing to use of several biomaterials for 3D printing. Although, each 3D printing process is based on different principles with their pros and cons.

Scaffold design is governed by pore size, pore structure, and lay-down pattern as scaffold architecture. However, each of them contributes significantly to the scaffold's desired output functions, i.e., mechanical properties and other derivative properties [50]. The porosity plays a leading role in architecture design and the desired biomechanical outcome of the scaffolds. Another critical parameter for scaffold design is pore structure, i.e., interconnectivity between two or more pores. For bone tissue engineering, it is expected to have 40- 60% volumetric porosity for efficient nutrient transport, cell migration, and ECM formation [52]. The most critical issue that needs attention is to converse mechanical strength performance concerning the scaffold's porosity. Raising the porosity will deteriorate the scaffold's strength due to reducing the scaffold's density function [52] [204]. The scaffold should have two kinds of porosity. One is macro-porosity (pore size in a range of 50μm to 1000μm) liable for osteogenic outcomes, the strength of a structure, and second is micro-porosity (pore size<10μm) accountable for bone induce protein absorption, drug absorption, apatite formations, and ion exchanges [61],[205], [206]. It is also expected to have a decent pore structure. The ideal pore structure is entirely interconnectivity between all pores for cell attachment, migration, and vascularization [50]. In the conventional fabrication processes, the random distribution pores will never assure interconnection between the pores. Though, there is always a debate for the exact definition of porosity dimensions and interconnected pore size dimensions (size in between 15-50 μm) [50] [206], [207]. The architecture of the scaffold is an essential parameter in scaffold design. Various laydown patterns, along with porosity and pore size, directly impacted the mechanical strength of the scaffold [208]. The detailed study for architecture design has been presented in chapter no.3.

The proposed chapter will concentrate on 3D plotting of various ceramic biomaterial composites and testing, followed by results, discussion, and conclusion.

4.2 Materials and Method
4.2.1 Materials

Tri calcium phosphate (β-TCP) [$Ca_3(PO_4)_2$] particle size 15μm ± 5μm and Hydroxyapatite (HA) [$Ca_5(PO_4)_3(OH)$] particle size 15μm ± 5μm is acquired from MEDICOAT®, France. Polyvinyl alcohol (PVA) [$(C_2H_4O)_x$] molecular weight 44.053 g/mol is procured from Fisher Scientific, India. Aluminium oxide [Al_2O_3] particle size 50 nm is acquired from Sigma Aldrich. Magnesium oxide (MgO) and Zirconium dioxide [ZrO_2] particle size 11-39 μm are acquired from Loba Chemie, India.

4.2.2 3D printing of ceramic biomaterials

Although the material's particle size is fine, all the materials are still sieved through a mesh size no # 500 as per the ASTM E11 standard to remove chunks. To assure the uniform particle size of less than 25 μm. Afterward, 20 grams of each proposed composite was prepared by adding 20 % of HA, 10 % of Al_2O_3, MgO, and ZrO_2 in β-TCP to form a four different composition categorized as the case I (20 % HA+β-TCP), case II (10 % Al_2O_3+β-TCP), case III (10 % MgO +β-TCP), and case IV (10 % ZrO_2+β-TCP). PVA binder solution has been prepared as per the procedure established by Sapkal et al. [40] and explain in brief. 3 grams of PVA powder is added to 37 grams of distilled water and stirred for 6 hours or until the transparent viscous solution is formed. The binder is then filtered through the Whatman® grade 1 filter paper with a pore size of 11 μm to remove suspended particles. Slurry with uniform viscosity has been formed by adding less than 40 Wt. % of binder in the composite powder as per requirement. The slurry is then loaded to 3D- Bioplotter® (Developer series, Envision TEC, Germany), an extrusion-based printing process. It comprises X-Y moving arms and Z-direction moving printing head. The air pressure is applied to a low-temperature printing head to exert pressure on the syringe cartridge, having a 400 µm nozzle at another end. The scaffold's robust CAD model with dimension 10×10×5 mm was designed on CREO® parametric design software by PTC, USA. The model is imported into Bioplotter RP software supplied by EnvisionTEC for uniform slicing and virtual mounting on the platform. The slices of uniform thickness 320 µm were selected, and a total of 15 slices were decided. The most practical and feasible 0^0-90^0 laydown pattern of the strand was decided for the scaffold. The machine's necessary operating parameter is controlled by another Visual machine software supplied by a Bioplotter manufacturer.

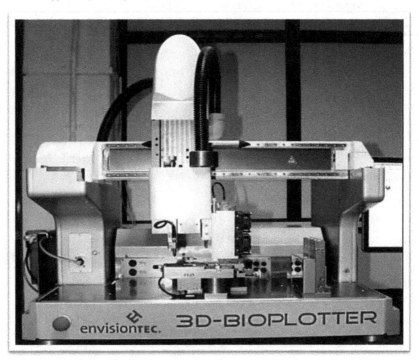

Figure 4.1 3D- Bioplotter system

4.2.2 Printability of biomaterials

The printability of slurry was an important issue, especially in extrusion-based printing. The slurry was dense enough to flow out of the nozzle and, at the same time, must retail the shape after printing. The initial trials were run for deciding the print conformity for fiber deposition at different pressure, print speed, nozzle height, and other related manufacturing criteria. Several experiments were run to decide the printing parameters for Case I. The printing speed is varied from 5 mm/s, 8 mm/s, 10mm/s, and 12 mm/s. The continue strand without deformability has been obtained at 10mm/s speed with dispensing pressure of 3.5 bar. Each of the parameters mentioned in table 4.1 was obtained after the number of experiments on each combination. The pre and post-flow delays were mentioned at 0.3 sec and 0.1 sec for material to flow and have proper bonding of strand with the previous layer before the printing process is completed. Before the printing of the new layer, the printer was kept on hold for 10 sec to give the time to settle down the printed layer. The printed scaffold is then sintered in a microwave furnace at 1200 °C for 30 min.

Table 4. 1 Printing parameter for ceramic biomaterial for present study

Parameters	Case I	Case II	Case III	Case IV
Printing Speed	10mm/s	15mm/s	12mm/s	8mm/s
dispense pressure	3.5 Bar	2.5 Bar	2.5 Bar	3.6 Bar
Temperature	20 °C	15 °C	15 °C	23 °C
Hold between each layer	10 Sec	10Sec	10 Sec	10 Sec
Pre flow delay	0.3 Sec	0.3 Sec	0.3 Sec	0.3 Sec
Post flow delay	0.1 sec	0.1 sec	0.1 sec	0.1 sec

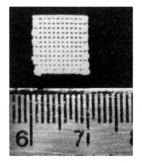 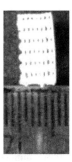

Figure 4.2 3D printed TCP: HA scaffold

4.2.3 Sintering of scaffold:

The 3D printed ceramic scaffold needs post-processing in the form of sintering for improvisation in mechanical strength. In the study, a microwave sintering furnace (MWS) is used for rapid sintering. Volumetric sintering is accumulated in microwave sintering with a high heating rate and low holding time than conventional sintering (CS). In conventional sintering, surface heating is provided at a slower rate along with prolonged holding or dwell time to get better and uniform sintering[176], [209], [210]. The scaffold is surrounded by susceptor-like Silicon carbide encapsulated by alumina brick are placed inside the microwave furnace. The sintering cycle followed, from room temperature (R_T) to 350^0C manual heating with a power supply of 200 Watt, after 350- 1200 ^0C heating rate provided is 15 ^0C/Min and dwell at sintered temperature (Ts) for 30 Min followed by standard furnace cooling.

4.2.4 Characterization of the composite scaffold

After the scaffold fabrication and thermal processing, it was tested for three different spectacles. The first is about physical and mechanical properties includes porosity, shrinkage, density, and compressive strength. Second, metallurgical characteristics comprise scanning electron microscopy (SEM), X-ray diffraction (XRD), Fourier transform infrared spectroscopy (FTIR) analysis. Last, the biological physiognomies contain cytotoxicity, drug delivery, and degradation study.

4.2.5 Porosity and density analysis

The relative density and porosity of the scaffold are measured based on Archimedes' principle using water as an immersing medium. The relative density is calculated by equation (i), and porosity is calculated by equation (ii) as below:

$$Relative\ Density = \frac{Bulk\ Density}{Theriotical\ Density} \quad \dots\dots\dots\dots(i)$$

$$Apparent\ Porosity\ (\%) = \frac{vp}{V} \quad \dots\dots\dots\dots\dots\dots(ii)$$

Where,

V (Volume of sample) = (W_3-W_1)/ density of water (~1.0 g/cc)

vp (Volume of pores) = (W_2-W_3)/density of water

W_1= Weight of sample immersed in water after detoxifying

W_2= Weight of sample along with water inside the sample

W_3= dry weight of a sample

Bulk or Archimedes density = (W$_3$)/ V

The theoretical density needed for relative density was calculated by the rule of mixture for the composite. The porosity of the green scaffold was calculated using equation three [189][211] in brief, represented in Figure 4.3. The porosity of scaffold for bone tissue engineering is approx. 40-60 %, accordingly, alteration in the distance between the strand was used to decide the pore size, as shown in table 4.2. From the theoretical calculations, it has been clear that the approx. 50 % of porosity can be achieved with a strand distance of 800 µm. Hence for all the cases, the distance between strands was kept the same.

$$p = 1 - \frac{\pi d_1^2}{4 d_2 d_3} \qquad \text{(iii)}$$

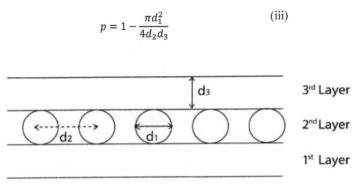

Figure 4. 3 Pore size alteration for desired porosity.

Table 4. 2 Theoretical Porosity calculation of scaffold

Theoretical Porosity							
d$_1$(strand dia.) (µm)	400	400	400	400	400	400	
d$_2$ (distance between strand) (µm)	500	600	700	800	900	1000	
d$_3$ (layer thickness) (µm)	320	320	320	320	320	320	
Porosity (%)	21.46	34.55	43.90	**50.91**	56.37	60.73	

4.2.6 Shrinkage

Sintering is a post-processing tool for enhancing mechanical strength, but it will also cause the shrinking of scaffolds. The pre-sintered scaffold shows a dissimilarity in dimensions after sintering refers to shrinkage. Although granule coalescence can cause shrinkage during the printing process, in this study, null hypotheses were made for such cases, and shrinkage only after sintering was considered. [61].

4.2.7 Compressive strength

A uniaxial compressive test was performed on a sintered scaffold for mechanical property evaluation. A Servo hydraulic universal testing machine set up with a crosshead speed of 0.65 mm/min at room condition is implemented for testing. Compressive strength is calculated by using maximum load at failure acted on the initial area.

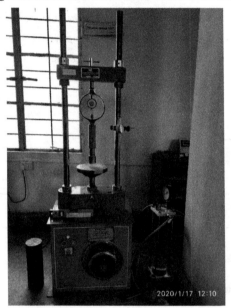

Figure 4.4 Compression testing setup

4.2.8 Scanning Electron Microscopy (SEM)

Sintered scaffold morphology was analyzed by scanning electron microscopy. Samples were coated with gold-palladium using JOEL JFC 1600 Auto beautiful coater from Japan and were mounted on aluminum stud with double adhesive tape. Images were scanned under different magnifications using the JOEL-6380A scanning electron microscope with the magnification at 27X, 50X, and 100X range.

4.2.9 X-Ray Diffraction (XRD) analysis

To analyze the effect of the sintering process on the physical structure of composite, the X-ray diffraction (XRD) analysis was performed. Tests were carried out with raw composite material and sintered composite materials. The sample was scanned from the range of 10^0 to 80^0, 2θ with a continuous scan rate of 0.0017, scan step time of

10.30 s with copper ray tube operated at 45KV and 40 mA. The fine crystal powder sample was placed on a slide under the X-ray source for analysis.

4.2.10 Fourier Transform Infrared Spectroscopy (FTIR) analysis.

Fourier transform infrared spectroscopy analysis of sintered scaffolds was carried out using Nicolet™ iS™5 Spectrometerwith a range of 4000–400 cm^{-1} from Thermo Scientific (Waltham, MA, USA). Infrared absorbance spectra of sintered ceramic composite materials and raw powder were recorded.

4.2.11 Biological characterization of the composite scaffold

After the achievement of mechanical and metallurgical desired properties, the next critical stage is biological evaluation. It may include but is not limited to cytocompatibility testing, drug delivery, degradation, etc. The cytocompatibility refers to the level of toxicity of material with a particular cell line. In BTE, such cytotoxicity will need to evaluate with the osteoblast cell line responsible for bone regeneration. In the proposed study, a human osteosarcoma cell line refers as MG63 is used for analysis. The cell line is procured from the National Center for Cell Sciences (NCCS) Pune, Maharashtra State, India. The cells are passaged as per the standard protocol prescribed by American Type Culture Collection (ATCC) for the adherent cell line. After receiving the cells from NCCS and achieving the confluence, more than 80 % of the cells are trypsinized with 0.05% trypsin and 0.04 % EDTA (for increasing the enzymatic action of trypsin solution.) followed by 15 min incubation. To stop trypsinization equal amount of cultured media is added to the solution. Centrifugation action was performed at 1000 RPM for 15 min. The supernatant was discarded, and cells were resuspended with the complete fresh medium in another T25 flask. The cell counting was performed with Automatic cell counter Countess™ II FL supplied by ThermoFisher Scientific USA as per the protocol. The complete culture media for the MG63 cell line was prepared with DMEM (Dulbecco's modified eagle medium), 25 µl/ml streptomycin, 10 µl/ml penicillin, 10 % heat-inactivated fetal bovine serum, and 25 µg/ml amphotericin B [75] [49]. After every 4-5 days and achieving confluence, the cells were passage into multiple flasks. More than 90% of viable cells were used for further study.

4.2.11.1 Cytotoxicity:

The material compatibility with cell line accessed by MTT [3-(4,5-dimethyl-2-thiazolyl)-2,5-diphenyl- 2H tetrazolium bromide] staining as per ISO10993-5:2009. Cell concentration with 3×10^4 cells/ml was seeded on a scaffold (5×5×2.5mm) specially prepared for MTT assay. The cell-laden scaffold was put in 10µl of MTT followed by 4 hours incubation at 37 ^{0}C for 24 and 48-hour compatibility testing. 100 µl of MTT solution is added in the presence, and the absence of scaffold in 24 well plates and cell metabolic activity were access in presence after 24 and 48 hours. After 4 hours of incubation, samples were placed into a new well plate, and 1ml of solubilizer (10% Triton X-100, 0.1N HCl, and isopropanol) was added to each well to dissolve the formazan crystals. The absorbance was measured at 570 nm using a microplate reader (Multiskan™ FL microplate photometer, Thermo Fisher Scientific USA). The absorbance of wells containing only complete culture media without scaffold is considered 100 % viable and used as a control for comparison. The relative growth rate (RGR) [67] was calculated by equation (iv).

$$RGR = \frac{Experimental\ group\ OD}{Control\ group\ OD} X100 \qquad \text{(iv)}$$

The result is then signified by using paired student T-test. The P-value obtained is less than 0.05, which shows the significant effect of the study. The data for statistical analysis is shown in Annexure IV.

4.2.11.2 Drug delivery:

The drug-laden scaffold improved their functionality for various disease treatment like osteomyelitis, TB arthritis etc. [67][70][135][47][212][213][214][215][199]. It gave the vigorous benefits of local drug concentration at the desired level for the required time and developed a broad interest in utilizing scaffold for its drug delivery functionality. In the present study, Vancomycin, an antibiotic used for osteomyelitis, was analyzed for drug kinetic study. The scaffold fabrication process employed will degrade the activity of the drug. Hence, the promising method for drug amalgamation is "impregnation" used in the study. Vancomycin solution at a concentration of 20 mg/ml was prepared in deionized water. The scaffold (5×5×2.5 mm) was 3D printed, followed by microwave sintering, immersed into the drug solution overnight at 37 ^{0}C in the presence of 5 % CO_2 in the incubator, and further analyzed for drug elution. Drug-loaded scaffolds were immersed individually in 10 ml PBS (pH 7.4) at 37 °C. A volume of 10 ml of PBS was chosen with the available previous literature, volume for significant immersion of scaffold, and approximate serum volume was chosen to approximate the volume of serum that would surround the scaffold packed into the dead space following bone debridement [76]. The elution medium was replaced after every 24 hours for the first five days, then 48 hours for the rest study. The aliquots were analyzed in a UV spectrophotometer for drug concentration at a wavelength of 280 nm. The calibration curve was generated using solutions with vancomycin concentration in the range of 0.5–100 (mg/ml), where the linear relationship of absorbance and concentration was obtained[76]. The study was performed for a total of 30 days.

4.2.11.3 *In Vitro* degradation testing:

To investigate the scaffold's degradation ability, each scaffold was incubated in DMEM supplemented with 10 % FBS at 37 °C and 5 % CO_2 chamber to simulate a living organism's environment. The initial weight was noted as W_O. The scaffold was removed after 1, 3, 5, 7, 14, and 21 days intervals, rinsed three times with deionized water to remove the ions and dried at 120 °C overnight, and the final weight of the sample (W_t) was measured. Weight loss for each day was calculated by using three samples for each time interval. The medium was changed after every alternate day to avoid contamination and saturation of released ions during the degradation process.

4.3 Result and discussion:
4.3.1 Physical and mechanical testing:

The scaffold was fabricated with a 10×10×5 mm dimension, and after sintering, the measured dimensions were less than the design. The average volume obtained after sintering was 423 ± 12.43 mm^3 for a case I, 409 ± 0.038 mm^3 for case II, 419 ± 0.013 mm^3, and 0.399 ± 0.012 mm^3 for case IV (Table 4.3), which account volumetric shrinkage 10.244 ± 3.740, 18.281 ± 7.665, 46.157 ± 2636, and 20.145 ± 2.446 respectively. Approximate similar results were noted in the previous literature [49] [61]. The shrinkage is a cooperative result of diffusion of matrix materials in the composite and evaporation of binder entrapped between the material molecules. The relative density measured as per

Archimedes' principle was found in the sequence of Case IV > Case I > Case II > Case III. These results are in correlation with the density of each composite.

Microwave sintering provides volumetric sintering essential for uniform heating and grain size formation [210], [216]. In microwave sintering, high heating rates and low holding time is advisable, resulting in rapid post-processing in comparison with the standard surface heating and sintering process [86], [209], [217]–[223]. The resulted percentage porosity at a range of 33.47 ± 0.981 to 59.199 ± 8.561 has been observed, which can satisfy the porosity requirement for bone tissue engineering applications [39], [40], [75], [85]. The compressive strength attained in all the cases is more than that of trabecular bone [224]. Sapkal et al. reported a compressive strength of 14.407 MPa, 51.06 % of porosity, for 20 % HA+ β-TCP when sintered in convectional sintering furnace 1400 °C [75]. The strength of 41.673 ± 5.247 MPa with 45.625 ± 5.071 % porous structure achieved with microwave sintering. It was assimilating the importance of microwave sintering in balancing strength, porosity, time, and energy saving.

Table 4.3 Parameters studied on the 3D printed sintered scaffold.

Composite	Width (mm)	Length (mm)	Height (mm)	Volume (mm^3)	Relative density	Shrinkage %	Porosity by ASTM B962-15	Strength (MPa)
Case-I (20 % HA +β TCP)	9.769 ±0.105	9.641 ±0.089	4.763 ±0.107	0.449 ±0.019	1.563 ± 0.174	10.244 ± 3.740	45.625 ±5.071	41.673 ±5.247
Case II (10%Al$_2$O$_3$+ β TCP)	9.512 ±0.256	9.604 ±0.258	4.464 ±0.181	0.409 ±0.038	0.862 ± 0.025	18.281 ± 7.665	33.476 ±0.981	60.794 ±5.228
Case III (10% MgO+β TCP)	9.698 ±0.121	9.855 ±0.123	4.388 ±0.190	0.419 ±0.013	0.536 ± 0.033	16.157 ± 2.636	47.676 ±2.925	51.839 ±8.744
Case IV (10% ZrO2+β TCP)	9.560 ±0.098	9.606 ±0.044	4.347 ±0.044	0.399 ±0.012	1.927 ± 0279	20.145 ± 2.446	59.199 ±8.561	66.900 ±1.822

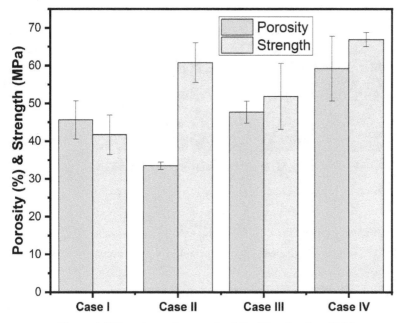

Figure 4. 5 Porosity and strength of the 3D printed scaffold

4.3.2 Phase assemblage, morphology, and compositional analysis:

Sintering effects widely on metallurgical properties like phase, morphology, and composition change. This was evaluated with SEM, XRD, and FTIR. A scanning electron microscope was used for the morphological study of the scaffold. The average stand diameter and pore size were observed 224.53 ± 16.96 μm and 667.27 ± 17.81 μm, respectively for case I. The drop in strand diameter is approximate 43.86 %, and in pore size, approximately 16.59 % has been observed as a sintering effect for the case I. For cases II & III, the pore size observed is 687.12 μm and 662.88 μm, respectively. For case IV, it is 592.04 μm. (Figure 4.6).

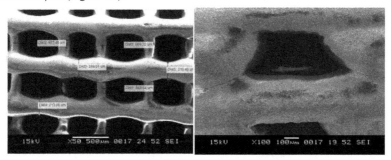

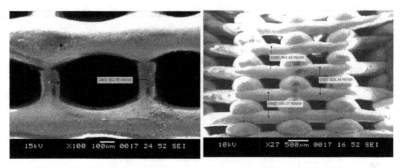

Figure 4.6 SEM showing the morphology of pore and strand

X-ray diffraction (XRD) was used to identify phase change due to high-temperature sintering. The picks obtained for sintered material are compared with the raw powder. Figure 4.7 shows the XRD profile for as received powder samples (raw powder) and 1200 ^{0}C microwave sintered powder. The profile does not accumulate any significant change in composition for all the cases.

FTIR spectrum shows the peaks at 589 cm^{-1} and 635 cm^{-1} are for the triply degenerate bending vibration of P_4^3 bonding. Sharp edge 571 cm^{-1} and 603.85 cm^{-1} is due to the presence of P_4^3 in β- TCP. No significant variation has been observed in spectra for a raw and sintered sample, as shown in Figure 4.8.

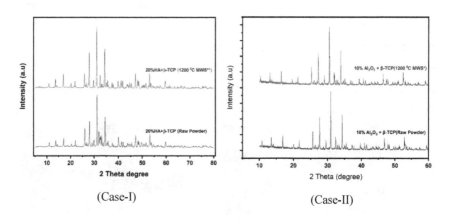

(Case-I) (Case-II)

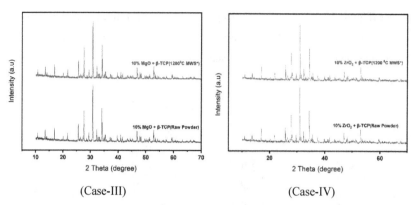

(Case-III)　　　　　　　　　　(Case-IV)

Figure 4.7 XRD profile of raw powder and sample sintered at 1200 ⁰C in microwave sintering.

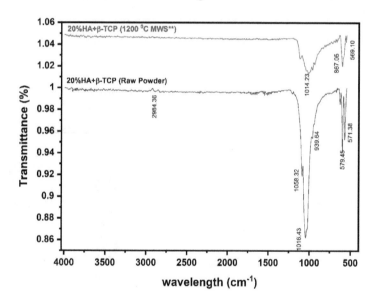

Figure 4.8 FTIR Spectra for raw powder and sintered powder at 1200 ⁰C.

4.3.3 Biological evaluation:

The scaffold, after the mechanical and phase transformation, compositional analysis was analyzed for its cytocompatibility, drug elution, and degradation. The cytocompatibility was checked with the MG 63 cell line. Cell metabolic activity with more than 80 % is considered compatible. Whereas if viability is less than 80 %, then the material is considered toxic. None of the composites has shown any toxic nature for the cell line (Figure 4.9). The statistical analysis to find the significance of the study was conducted through Studen T-test. The P-value obtained through this analysis is p value< 0.05, representing the significance of the study.

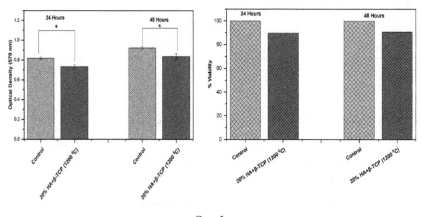

Case I

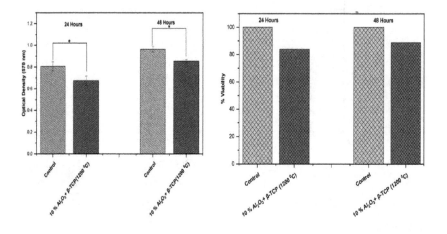

(Case-II)

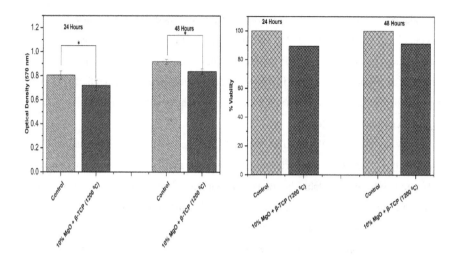

Case III

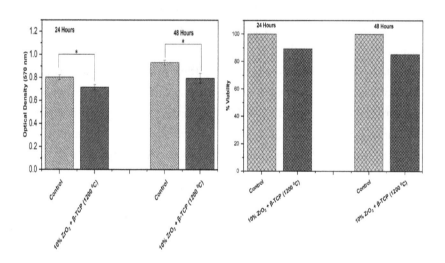

Case IV

**Figure 4.9 24 and 48-hour cytotoxicity analysis of composite material
(* p-value <0.05 showing the significance of the study)**

Change in weight of scaffold when subjected in contact with the body fluid in our study DMEM + 10 % FBS concerning the scaffold's dry weight will give a scaffold degradation profile. (Figure 4.10) It was seen that in this case, I show slow and steady degradation, which might be due to 20 % HA reinforced in the composite. HA is osteoinductive, which makes it favorable for bone tissue engineering. Still, at the same time, the degradation rate of HA is prolonged that something refers to negligible by many researchers [225]. On the contrary, another calcium phosphate material like β/α TCP has a good degradation profile.

While in case II (10 % Al_2O_3 + β TCP) has shown functional degradation, Case I due to only 10 % Al_2O_3 is incorporated in the composite matrix. However, Aluminum oxide is bioinert and non-degradable, but its assimilation provides stability to the scaffold, which results in control over the weight loss. In case III, magnesium oxide shows a higher degradation rate than any other material because magnesium itself holds the degradation characteristics, representing the higher degradation than any other composite. Zirconium dioxide has a compressive strength of 2000 MPa and a 5.68 gm/cc density, the highest in biomaterials. ZrO_2 is one of the most robust and hardest materials, making it hostile for application where degradation is not required. (Figure 4.10)

Drug release can be achieved due to two reasons. The first is the diffusion of drug molecules, and the second is the degradation of biomaterials. (Figure 4.11) Considering these two facts, HA and MgO have a similar drug delivery rate because both materials are biodegradable and contribute more to drug release. Simultaneously, the other two materials are bioinert and result in a slow degradation rate. It will open up the new scaffold application doors, especially for bone infection, inflammation, and other diseases. The drug or BMP-laden scaffold not only improves the functionality but also helps in effective treatment management.

The small amount amalgamation of material like Al_2O_3 or ZrO_2 helps to improve the mechanical stability and also results in prolonging drug elusion as per the result obtained. During the impregnation method, the drug is entrapped inside two materials molecules' pores and absorbed by the material itself. When it comes in contact with body fluid, this drug-loaded scaffold starts to release the drug. The rate of drug release is directly proportional to the combined effect of diffusion and degradation of materials. As the degradation does not take place for the bioinert materials, the slow drug release is obtained. This is the reason that we got a slow release in cases II and IV. On the contrary, for the case I and III, the degradation is higher than the other two compounds.

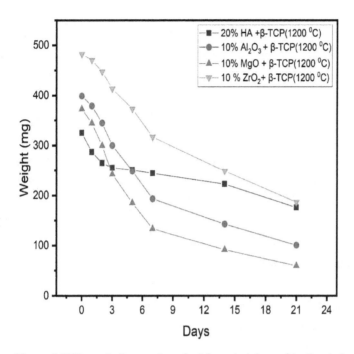

Figure 4.10 Degradation contour for biomaterials used in the study

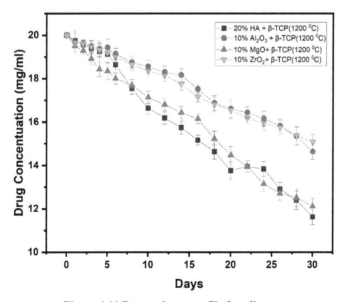

Figure 4.11 Drug release profile for all cases

4.4 Conclusion:

Ceramic biomaterials are widely used for bone tissue regeneration for three decades. However, the optimum biomaterials and their combination is still a field of research. Case I (20% HA + -TCP), Case II (10% Al2O3 + -TCP), Case III (10% MgO + -TCP), and Case IV (10% Zro2 + -TCP) were tested for physiological, mechanical, Phase assemblage, morphology, and compositional analysis, as well as biological physiognomies. The decision-making parameters in our study are porosity, compressive strength, drug elution, and degradation. Shrinkage is not considered a decision-making parameter. It is a highly repeatable and unavoidable defect that can be compensated by scaling the initial CAD model before printing. The highest porosity and compressive strength were obtained in IV, i.e., 10 % ZrO_2 + β-TCP because zirconia has the highest compressive strength than other ceramics. However, its bioinert nature restricted its utilization in tissue engineering. A small and optimum amount of ZrO_2 can be used in implants and open the door to new research. Similarly, in case II (10 % Al_2O_3 + β-TCP), it also reveals good strength and adequate porosity, but the slow drug liberation and bioinert nature make it substandard for tissue engineering application.

The compressive strength for the case I (20 % HA + β-TCP) and III (10 % MgO + β-TCP) is 41.67 and 51.83 MPa. They also show excellent characteristics during drug release. Being a fifth important element of the body and degradable, MgO is now considered in scaffold for regeneration. With this research work, one more application of MgO as a drug delivery vehicle will take attention. It is hard to regulate the degradation rate of ceramic material as compared with a polymeric material. Nevertheless, a small amount of material modification in the composite can enhance degradation and improve its utilization.

CHAPTER 5: CRITICAL ANALYSIS OF THE SINTERING OF CERAMIC BIOMATERIALS.

5.1 Introduction

In the last few decades, significant efforts were made to develop materials with better biocompatibility, superior mechanical and functional properties. With the advancement in technology, the challenges in patient-specific or customization in materials are conceivable. Biomaterial provides a three-dimensional template referred to as a scaffold to act as a synthetic extracellular matrix (ECM) for tissue regeneration and drug delivery [220]. The biomaterial could be polymer, ceramic, metal, or composite as per need of tissue interest or desired tissue responses. For bone tissue, renaissance ceramic biomaterials are the first choice of researchers and clinicians. The ceramic biomaterial was employed as a grafting medium for more than a century due to its mineral phase similarity with natural bone. Amongst the different bio-ceramic materials, hydroxyapatite shows a promising result in hard tissue engineering and makes it suitable only for non-load bearing areas for implantation [176]. Hydroxyapatite (HA) has good mechanical strength and bioactivity but lacks degradation due to the Ca/P ratio equal to 1.67. However, tricalcium phosphate (α or β phase) shows promising results along with bioactivity, osteointegration, and bio-degradation as an effect of Ca/P ratio 1.5 [220]. There is a wide range of scaffold fabrication processes, and each of them retains its advantages and disadvantages. The review of bioceramic material fabrication demonstrates each process's achievability, specifically in bone tissue engineering [4]. None of the fabrication processes for ceramic scaffold fabrication influences the mechanical strength equivalent to trabecular bone. It always needs post-fabrication maneuvers either in the form of crosslinking: mostly for ceramic and polymeric composite [226], [227] or sintering: the heat gradient process performed for material property enhancement without liquefaction [38], [108], [176], [218], [228]–[230]. Out of these two, the most common treatment for ceramic scaffold properties improvisation is sintering. There are several methods of sintering. Conventional sintering, Microwave sintering, Spark Plasma sintering, etc., are broadly used for ceramic materials. Conventional sintering occurs when the heat is provided to the outer surface of the sample and allows it to travel inside with the slow temperature gradient. Champion reviewed the sintering process related to calcium phosphate ceramic which includes solid-state pressure less sintering referred to as conventional sintering, two-stage sintering (TSS), and another advanced sintering process such as hot pressing (HP), hot isostatic pressing (HIP), microwave sintering (MWS) and sparks plasma sintering (SPS) and found higher densification, fine grains, higher strength can be achieved with advance sintering process [231]. Makireddi et al. show the importance of a slow heating rate for ceramic material processing in a conventional sintering muffle furnace and reported high strength and high hardness for a slower heating rate when sintered for two-step sintering [232]. Ghasali et al. did a comparative study of microwave and spark plasma sintering. During experimentation, he found 51.3% relative density in MWS while fully dense ceramic composite in SPS. He also revealed higher mechanical strength of the SPS sample as compare with MWS samples [223]. Lin et.al; worked on two-stage conventional sintering process briefly t_1=1050 ^{0}C for 0 hours and t_2= 950 ^{0}C for 20 hours. His experimental research represents improved fracture toughness, hardness, and relative density by 57 %, 12 %, and ~ 99.02 %, respectively [233]. Yin et al. performed a comparative study for one-stage and two-stage MWS on ceramic materials. In his material, he claims that single-stage MWS is always better than two-stage MWS because it controls grain growth and whisker formation [234]. Veljovic et al. work precisely with bioceramic material and found a decrease in grain size at the nano level and increase in toughness when bioceramic material is microwave sintered at two stages, along with saving in sintering cycle time and power in comparison with conventional sintering process [230]. Tarafder et al. work on TCP doping with MgO and SrO, followed by microwave sintering, and noted a significant improvement in mechanical strength due to higher densification achieved by volumetric heating by MWS [175]. The ideal scaffold for bone tissue engineering required macro and microporosity for effective cell migration, vascularization, cell biomaterial attachment, impregnation of biological fluid, nutrient delivery, and greater surface area [235]. However, some fabrication processes like additive manufacturing contribute to marginal control over the porosity, pore size, and interconnectivity in green samples. Contrarily, post-processing, as discussed above, results in a compromise with porosity and pore size but increased mechanical strength due to higher densification. Besides that, there is phase transformation from HA to β-TCP [176] [236]; β-TCP to α-TCP [38] if temperature increases above 1250 ^{0}C. The mechanical strength and porosity are inversely proportional, along with temperature and sintering conditions. In present work, we are trying to evaluate and compare the conventional and microwave sintering for its mechanical and metallurgical properties for βTC + HA using the compression pellet fabrication process.

5.2 Materials:

Tri calcium phosphate (β-TCP) [$Ca_3(PO_4)_2$] particle size 15μm ± 5μm, Hydroxyapatite (HA) [$Ca_5(PO_4)_3(OH)$] particle size 15μm ± 5μm are acquired from MEDICOAT®, France. The Composite of different matric ratios was selected as per the research experience for finite element analysis results obtained for bone tissue engineering previously by us [208]. The ceramic powder was mixed by ball milling for 8 hours at 400 RPM, and the weight ratio of ball to powder is 10:1. Polyvinyl alcohol (PVA) [$(C2H4O)x$] molecular weight 44.053 g/mol is procured from Fisher Scientific, India, used as a binder for fabricating the pellets in different ratios.

5.3 Experimental:

5.3.1 Binder preparation:

Polyvinyl alcohol (PVA) binder solution has been prepared by adding PVA to deionized water at 1, 2, 3, 4, 5, 6, and 7 wt % continuous stirrers at medium speed for 10 hours till a transparent viscous solution has been formed. The binder is then gravitationally filtered through the Whatman® grade 1 filter paper with a pore size of 11 μm to remove suspended particles. Figure 5.1 depicts the various binder concentration solutions used in the experiment.

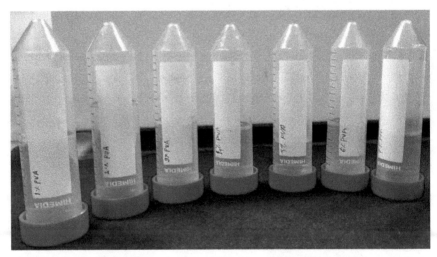

Figure 5.1 PVA binder solution (1 to 7 Wt % concentration from left to right)

5.3.2 Bio-ceramic composite pellet fabrication:

The composite powder was placed inside cylindrical steel die with 10 mm diameter and pressed uniaxially using a hydraulic pellet press. Due to the change in binder concentration in bioceramic slurry, the uniaxial pressure value needs to change for each condition. The good pellet is considered with two thoughts; firstly, the mixture of composite and binder should not be thin slurry to make it impossible to fabricate pellets. Secondly, no crack and deformities should be noticeable in green pellets. The pellets are then processed for conventional and microwave sintering.

5.3.3 Convectional sintering (CS):

The pellets were sintered in conventional thermal heating furnaces (Okay Electric furnace India), as shown in Figure 5.2. The sintering cycle decided for all cases is brief: room temperature (T_R) to sintering temperature (T_S) heating rate is 5 oC/ min. The sample was kept on hold at T_s for 240 min, afterward standard furnace cooling until room temperature. Three different sintering temperature 1000, 1100, 1200 ^0C is designated for the study.

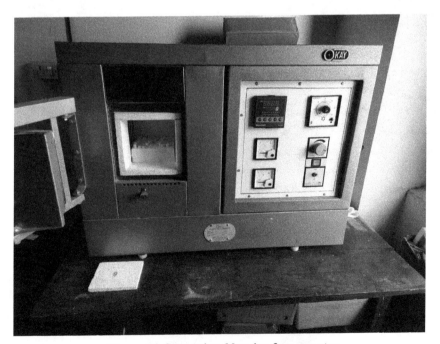

Figure 5.2 Convectional heating furnace setup

5.3.3 Microwave sintering (MWS):

Promising results in terms of mechanical strength and porosity obtained from convectional sintering are only compared with MWS samples sintered at T_s= 1200 °C. For MWS, three different heating rates (10, 15, 20 °C/min) and holding times (30 min) for the study have been decided. The threshold value for our microwave sintering furnace is 350 °C below, in which the power is supplied manually at a 200 Watt rate, and once the threshold value is reached, the furnace was shifted to pre-defined program mode.

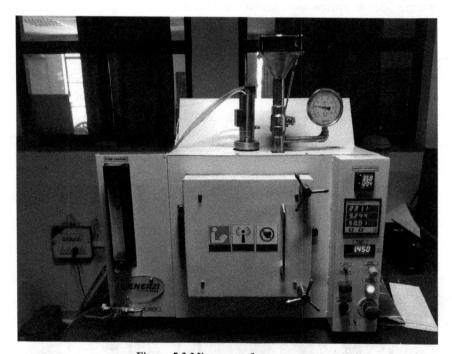

Figure 5.3 Microwave furnace setup

5.3.4 Density measurement:

The density was measured as per ASTM standard B962-15, which is based on the Archimedes principle using distilled water as an immersion medium and elucidate by researchers [41][231][223][209][237]. The bulk density of each sample was measured after convectional and microwave sintering with triplicate samples for each study. The Composite's theoretical density was calculated by the rule of the mixture using the densities of the individual components: β-TCP- 3.14, HA - 3.18, (all in g/cm³). The relative density can be obtained by the equation below:

$$Relative\ Density\ \%\ (\rho) = \frac{Bulk\ Density}{Therotical\ Density} \times 100 \qquad (v)$$

5.3.5 Porosity measurement:

The apparent porosity of each pellet after conventional and microwave sintering was measured and calculated by density difference by using the following formulas:

$$Porosity\ (\%) = \frac{(Theoretical\ density - Actual\ density)}{Theoretical\ Density} \times 100 \qquad (vi)$$

5.3.6 Shrinkage:

The pellet dimensions were measured before and after post-conventional and microwave sintering with the help of a digital Vernier caliper. The volumetric shrinkage was observed, and all the samples and data are represented as an average of triplicated samples. The overall volumetric shrinkage has been calculated.

5.3.7 Compressive strength measurement:

A uniaxial compression test was performed on a pellet using a hydraulic compression test machine with a spindle speed of 0.65mm/min, as shown in Figure 5.4. The result of the compression test was represented in Figure 5.7 and Annexure-II.

5.3.8 X-ray diffraction (XRD) analysis:

The Phase comparison of composite powder and residue of compression test were analyzed by XRD using Rigaku-D/Max-2500 diffractometer operated at 30 kV/200 mA using Cu Kα radiation (1.54056 Å). Data were collected at room temperature at a 2 mm/min scanning speed over a 2θ range of 10-80 °.

5.3.9 Fourier Transforms Infrared spectroscopy (FTIR) analysis:

Fourier transform infrared spectroscopy analysis of raw ceramic Composite and residue of sintered pellets after compression test was carried away using Nicolet™ iS™5 Spectrometer with a range of 4000–400 cm⁻¹ from Thermo Scientific (Waltham, MA, USA). Infrared absorbance spectra of sintered ceramic composite materials and raw powder were recorded.

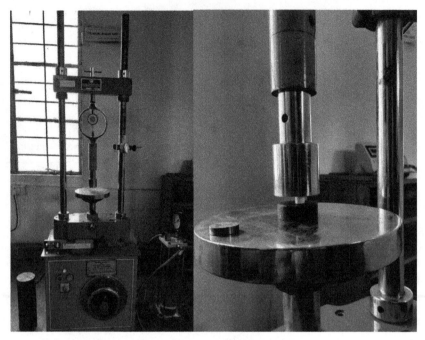

Figure 5.4 Compression test setup.

5.4 Results and Discussion:

5.4.1 Pelleting conditions:

The pellet was fabricated by pressing Composite inside the die uniaxially. The parameter that affects getting good pellets are PVA concentration, binder weight % used in slurry, and the pressure applied. Figure 5.5 represent the various applied load concerning binder concentration. From Figure 5.5, it is clear that the pressure applied is inversely proportional to binder concentration. A higher load can produce good pellets for low concentration but reduce the voids between the particles resulting reduction in porosity. However, optimum binder ratio and load can produce a good pellet, along with porosity, due to the evaporation of binder trapped inside the material particles. To get an excellent pellet for further study is only possible at certain PVA comprised in binder ratio and explain in Figure 5.6. The pellets with the right physical conditions.

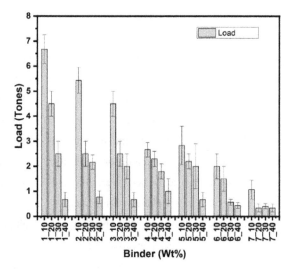

Figure 5.5 Applied pressure and binder concentration variation relationship

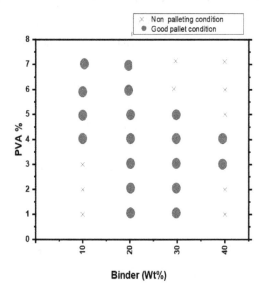

Figure 5.6 Good pellet condition at particular PVA wt. % in binder

5.4.2 Physical and Mechanical analysis:

The good pellets obtained as per requirements are further evaluated for different parameters like change in volume, density, porosity, volumetric shrinkage, and strength at

1000, 1100, 1200 °C (Annexure I & II). Figure 5.9 (a) gives the graphical representation of porosity change concerning binder concentration for different temperatures. It has been found that with an increase in sintering temperature, the porosity reduces as a result of shrinkage of samples. The pellets are then subjected to compressive strength measurement as per the protocol. Ideally, the L/D ratio for the cylindrical sample should be ≥2. However, it is less than two; it needs to multiply with correction factors per ASTM C39 standard to get the actual strength value. Figure 5.9 (b) shows the strength results for 1000, 1100, 1200 °C by conventional sintering. For tissue engineering applications, a balance between porosity and strength is obligatory. Hence, we need to create a standard ground comparison for both the desired properties, which are planed with the help of porosity ratio, strength ratio, and calculating worth factor. The worth factor is obtained by multiplying both the ratio. Figure 5.9(c) shows the graphical depiction of all the porosity and strength data, and accordingly, the best combination decided for microwave sintering are binder ratio:1_30, 2_20, 3_20, 4_40, 5_30, 6_10, and 7_10 (Annexure I & II). The heating rate for microwaves was varied from 10, 15, and 20 °C/min to decide the finest heating. Table 5.1 shows the strength value for each heating rate and found the highest strength values in 15 °C/min.

Further microwave sintering experiments were performed with 15 °C/min for 30 min hold at sintering temperature. Figure5.8 shows the graphical representation of porosity, strength for the best binder combination, while Figure 5.9 represents the porosity ratio, strength ratio, and a worth factor used as decision-making tools for getting the optimal combination through experimentations. The worth factor projection noticed that binder combination 1_30 shows the optimum values of 18.75 % of porosity, 90.453 ± 1.752 % relative density gives 41.67 MPa compressive strength more than that of cancellous bone [224].

Table 5.1 Microwave sintering heating rate and effect on strength

MWS Heating rate	Porosity	Strength
10 °C/min	22.095 ± 6.01	37.33 ± 7.23
15 °C/min	20.928 ± 5.17	41.66 ± 14.01
20 °C/min	26.995 ± 1.73	24.30 ± 3.55

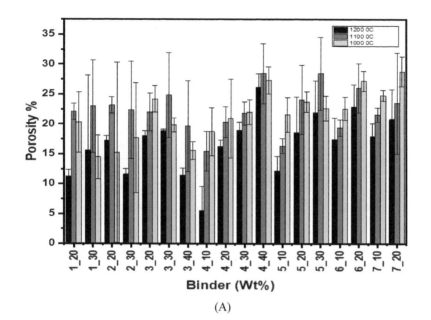

(A)

(B)

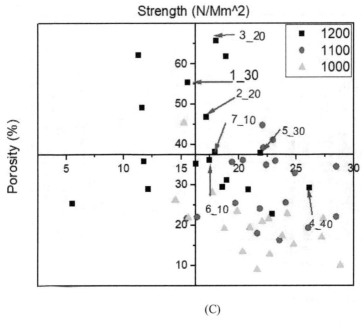

(C)

Figure 5.7 Mechanical properties representation for convectional sintered material. A) Change in porosity with binder ratio. B) change in the strength of pellet concerning binder formulation and temperature of sintering. C) the best binder formulation observed in all sintering cycles, i.e., 1000, 1100, 1200 0C.

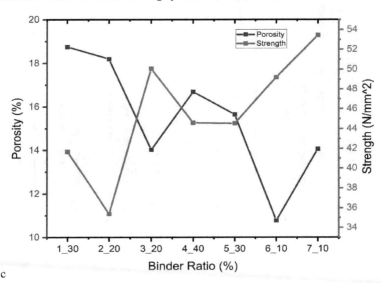

c

Figure 5. 8 Strength and porosity change graph for microwave sintering

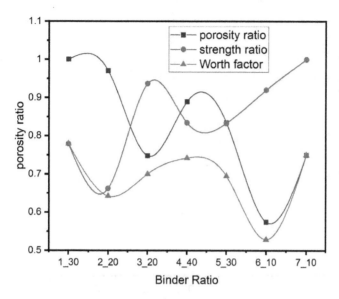

Figure 5.9 Worth factor projection

Worth factor projection used to decide the best suitable combination based conventional sintering process. The worth factor was calculated by simply multiplying the strength and porosity. This worthiness gives the optimum combination of the scaffold, which is further considered for microwave sintering. It helped minimize the experiments for the microwave sintering and reduce the time of the study.

5.4.3 Phase assemblage and compositional analysis:

XRD and FTIR study shows the effect of sintering temperature on metallurgical properties. The XRD contour for raw powder composite and conventional and microwave sintered powder was represented in Figure 5.10. Peak location for sintered 20 % HA + β TCP was in line with 20 % HA + β TCP in raw powder for 10-80 °. No phase change has been observed in XRD due to the high-temperature sintering of material and makes it safe for further investigation. FTIR characterization was performed to examine the effect of various sintering temperatures, composite bonds, and structure processes. The spectrum shows the pick and 589 cm^{-1} and 635 cm^{-1} are for the triply degenerate bending vibration of PO_4^3 bonding. Sharp edge 571 cm^{-1} and 603.85 cm^{-1} is due to the presence of PO_4^3 in β-TCP. No significant variation has been observed in spectra for as-prepared composite powder (raw powder) and sintered sample, as shown in Figure 5.11.

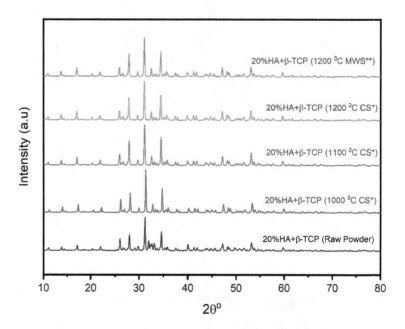

Figure 5.10 XRD plot for β-TCP + 20% HA

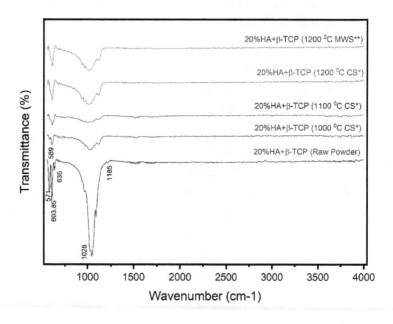

Figure 5.11 FTIR spectra for materials.

5.4.4 Cytocompatibility:

In Vitro, cytotoxicity was evaluated by MTT assay. The MTT assay shows the significant differences between 20 % HA+ β TCP sintered at various temperatures and methods concerning the control group during 24 hours and 48 hours of incubation. It appears that optical density and % viability increases with culture time, Figure 5.12. In, microwave sintered pellets have shown better results than conventional. Optical density for the MWS pellet at 1200 °C found approximate 8 and 12% increment for 24 hours and 48 hour incubation periods compared to control, respectively. It is noticeable that the convection sintering at 1200 °C for 4 hours and microwave sintering at 1200 °C for 30 min accelerates cell fate properties. The P-value obtained for the result is then signified by using paired student T-test. The P-value obtained is less than 0.05, which shows the significant effect of the study.

5.5 Conclusion:

The study concludes with the high impact of convectional and microwave sintering processes on the materials for their mechanical properties. The compressive strength of selected Composite (20 % HA + β-TCP) with binder ratio 1_30 was increased approximately 1.12_x at 1200 °C and 0.56_x at 1100 °C concerning sintering 1000 °C. The rise in porosity was also observed at the rate of 0.08_x at 1200 °C and 0.59_x at 1100 °C, according to results at 1000 °C. Shrinkage enhancement at rates of approximately 4.39_x at 1200 °C and 2.02_x at 1100 °C in connection with observation at 1000 °C. This increase in shrinkage represents the higher densification of samples at high temperatures. Conventional sintering is further compared with microwave sintering and originated with the rapid sintering of sample and saving in time and energy consumption suitably with convection sintering. The results concerning the growth in approx. 54.35_x for shrinkage, 0.21_x for porosity, 0.45_x in relative density but drop down to 24.75_x in compressive strength in MWS with a heating rate of 15 °C/min and dwell of 30 min. This will open up the field of rapid sintering combined with additive manufacturing for the fast delivery of biomaterial constructs to the clinical process.

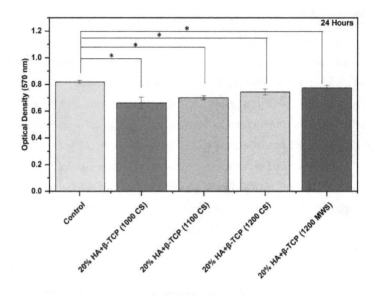

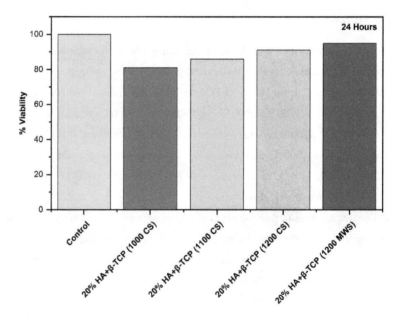

(A) 24 Hours cytotoxicity results

CHAPTER 6: CONCLUSION

- Contemporary technology in bio-engineering like image processing, computer-assisted manufacturing, and design additive manufacturing gives rise to customization in almost every medical application. Advancements in tissue engineering, material science, and other related fields make it possible to fabricate patient-specific scaffolds with desired compressive strength, porosity, and controlled degradation rate. Nevertheless, to date, 3D printed scaffold is looked at as a grafting medium only. The utilization of scaffold for two or more functions like multiple drugs is another exciting area of research.

- The next generation of research in tissue engineering is about the development of in-vitro biological model to study pathogenesis, treatment modality, and somehow new drug development. For these, we need a novel scaffold fabrication technology for rapid use. Additive manufacturing has come up with the advantages of zero complexity for the manufacturing of biomaterials. Microwave sintering and additive manufacturing are new approaches toward getting the speedy delivery of a scaffold.

- The simulation was helpful to understand the probable effect of using different material combinations. The result suggests that using a higher percentage of HA (up to 30%) in the composite will provide a favorable condition due to its mineral similarity with natural bone, osteoconductive, osteoinductive nature. Simultaneously, other materials like Al_2O_3, MgO, ZrO_2 can be incorporated only in small amounts, i.e., 10%. The lay down, or architecture complexity, increase the porosity due to providing more surface area to volume ratio and affecting the compressive strength of the scaffold. A balance between porosity and strength can be achieved virtually with the help of finite element simulation and help reduce the actual experimentation.

- The different cases considered for the experimental analysis are based on simulation results. Four different cases, namely case I (20%HA +β-TCP), Case II (10% Al_2O_3+β-TCP), Case III (10% MgO + β-TCP), and case IV (10% ZrO_2 + β-TCP), was evaluated for physical, mechanical, Phase assemblage and compositional analysis and biological parameters. The scaffold was sintered at 1200 °C in a microwave sintering furnace. No significant difference in XRD and FTIR has been found. It will represent that the phase and minerals after sintering remained the same as that of raw material. The lowest compressive strength was attained in case I (41.63 MPa), while case IV shows the highest strength value (66.91 MPa). This clarifies that the addition of different biomaterials in different combinations can regulate the strength. The degradation study represents the faster degradation in Case III than any other material, taking advantage of the Magnesium's corrosive property. The drug delivery analysis signifies the controlled and steady drug delivery in case I and case III. This is due to taking added advantages of diffusion of drug and degradation of materials.

- The most common route for the post-processing of ceramic material is sintering. However, conventional sintering is very time-consuming due to the slow heating rate and transmission of heat from the surface to inside, resulting in uneven heating of the scaffold. The microwave sintering provides volumetric heating at 3_X of heating rate and 24.75_X reduction in compressive strength. While the holding time in MWS is only 30 min, and convectional sintering is 240 min. These results show that the effective use of microwave sintering as compare with conventional sintering. The material sintered at different temperatures shows the cytocompatibility with MG 63 cell line, and no change in phase and composition has been observed.

CPSIA information can be obtained
at www.ICGtesting.com
Printed in the USA
LVHW021222160323
741693LV00041B/2093